TABLE OF CONTENTS

TABLE OF CONTENTS (continued)

TABLE OF CONTENTS (continued)

TABLE OF CONTENTS (continued)

TABLE OF CONTENTS (continued)

List of Appendixes

List of Tables

TABLE OF CONTENTS (continued)

List of Tables (continued)

List of Exhibits

List of Exhibits (continued)

TABLE OF CONTENTS (continued)

List of Exhibits (continued)

TABLE OF CONTENTS (continued)

List of Exhibits (continued)

TABLE OF CONTENTS (continued)

List of Exhibits (continued)

TABLE OF CONTENTS (continued)

List of Exhibits (continued)

TABLE OF CONTENTS (continued)

List of Exhibits (continued)

1. OVERVIEW OF PHYSICIAN EXAMINATION

1.1   The Role of the Physician in NHANES

Physicians function as mobile examination center (MEC) team members with the primary function of serving as the safety officer, as well as collecting blood pressure, heart rate, and pulse data. These measurements are the data source for reporting the national standard for blood pressure and heart rate from the NHANES. The American Heart Association blood pressure protocol is used, which results in standardized data collection across both MEC teams. The physician examination protocol, described in detail in Chapter 4, emphasizes the importance of following the protocol for the purpose of systematic, prioritized survey data collection.

The physician also serves as a resource in the support of the phlebotomy component. When SPs express concern about the blood draw either for themselves or their children, the physician can discuss the blood draw procedure with the SP, as well as promoting the benefit of the many tests that are reported.

Physicians play a role in the pubertal maturation section that is administered in the ACASI section of the MEC Interview to SPs aged 8-19. Before SPs under the age of 18 are assigned to the MEC Interview, a parent/guardian will be informed during the Automated Proxy Interview that his or her child will be asked questions about body development. Before the children are asked these questions, the parent or guardian's informed consent must be obtained during the proxy questionnaire. If the parent expresses reservations or concerns about these drawings, or other aspects of the pubertal maturation section, the MEC staff administering the proxy questionnaire offers the parent the opportunity to discuss the pubertal maturation section with the physician.

1.2   Medical Policy Regarding the Examination

The purpose of the NHANES study is to collect data on the health status of the United States population. The MEC is not a medical treatment facility, hence MEC physicians do not provide diagnoses or treatment of medical conditions. It is important to emphasize that treatment is **not** within the role of the

MEC physician, and any clinical findings that are of concern to physicians are documented and included in community practitioner referrals. In most instances, the examining physician will not be licensed within the state in which the examinations are being conducted. The liability insurance obtained for Westat physicians does not cover any type of treatment procedure except for medical emergency stabilization while awaiting the arrival of local paramedics.

The NHANES survey teams have neither control over, nor connection with, local health care systems. Any physician involvement beyond routine referral is ineffective and interferes with the purpose of the study. Referral of examinees is included in the MEC procedures for ethical reasons, although referral is not within the purpose of the study. Before SPs depart the MEC, they are provided with a Report of Findings that becomes available while they are in the MEC. They are provided a final report of all findings approximately 3 months after their MEC examination. These are in the form of written reports and they are mailed to the SPs.

1.2.1 Presence in MEC during MEC Examinations

Examinations do not occur in the MEC without the presence of a physician. Physicians report to the MEC at least 5 minutes before examinations are scheduled to begin. They leave the MEC only when all examination and interview protocol procedures have been completed and all SPs have left the MEC.

1.2.2 Response to Medical Emergencies

If an examinee becomes ill or disabled during the examination session, the physician renders only the level of care necessary to keep the examinee out of immediate danger. Arrangements are made to transport SPs to an appropriate medical facility. An ambulance is called if a potentially life threatening condition develops, or if indicated for any SP. Further details about medical emergencies are included in Chapter 6.

1.2.3 Maintenance of Emergency Equipment and Supplies

Physicians maintain emergency equipment and supplies for use in the MEC. They inventory supplies, restock supplies as needed, and ensure that all emergency equipment, medications, and supplies are current and in proper working order. Emergency procedures and supplies are described in detail in Chapter 6.

1.3 Physician Examination

The physician examination is described in detail in Chapter 3, Physician Protocol. The physician examination consists of:

- Heart rate on all SPs through 4 years of age. Radial pulse is counted on SPs from 5 years of age through age 7, and blood pressure and radial pulse are measured on all SPs aged 8 years and older.

- A discussion on the STD testing done on the survey and recruitment of male and female SPs aged 14-59 to self-collect a swab to test for Human Papillomavirus (HPV). The physician instructs the SP on how to obtain the specimen. The physicians instruct SPs on how to obtain their confidential STD test results via telephone.

- Medical referral generation -- physicians review data obtained during the MEC examination and, when indicated, they refer SPs to health care providers in the local community. Physicians are responsible for monitoring out-of-range data values as defined by the component protocols. If data values exceed predefined limits, the ISIS system flags these data for review. Physicians are responsible for discussing out-of-range values with SPs and making referrals to outside physicians if necessary. Physicians' procedures for managing referrals are described in Chapter 4.

1.4 Maintenance of Physician's Examination Room

Physicians are individually responsible for the maintenance of the physician's examination room and all equipment and supplies required for their examination. At the beginning of a stand, physicians inventory the required supplies and equipment. They prepare the examination room by opening and setting up all supplies and equipment needed for the physician examination. They determine that adequate supply levels are available and that all equipment is in proper working order. At the end of each examination session, physicians clean and properly store all equipment and restock supplies as needed. At the end of each stand, physicians inventory equipment and supplies and then pack up the equipment and supplies. Details about equipment maintenance and supplies are included in Chapter 2, Equipment and Supplies.

2. EQUIPMENT AND SUPPLIES

2.1 Description of Equipment and Supplies

The physician maintains, tracks, and orders all equipment and supplies necessary for the conduct of all aspects of the physician component, including:

- Blood pressure/pulse;

- HPV testing;

- Office supplies;

- Emergency management supplies; and

- OSHA bloodborne pathogen exposure forms and kit.

2.2 Inventory

For the purposes of inventory management, equipment is designated as nonconsumable items, and supplies are those items that are depleted throughout a stand and used on a daily basis. At the beginning and end of each stand, the physician will inventory all component-specific equipment and supplies. Supplies ordered from the warehouse by the previous team during teardown should be on site when the next team arrives to set up a new stand. Physicians will check all newly received supplies against the associated packing lists before incorporating them into the existing inventory. After reconciling the supplies, the physician will stock the exam room. Any needed items should be noted on the inventory list, reported to the chief technologist and to the MEC manager, and documented in the Unusual Field Occurrence (UFO) system.

2.3 Blood Pressure

Equipment is selected that meets the requirements for obtaining the required data and creates the best opportunity for minimal data collection error. All equipment is regularly subjected to quality control checks. Quality control procedures for physician equipment are described in detail in Chapter 8, Physician Equipment Quality Control.

2.3.1   Blood Pressure Equipment

- Baumanometer® calibrated mercury true gravity wall model sphygmomanometer;

- Baumanometer® calibrated mercury true gravity portable desk model sphygmomanometer (1);

- Baumanometer Calibrated V-Lok® cuffs with Latex Inflation Bulb, Air-Flo Control Valve in four sizes: child, adult, large adult, and thigh;

- Littman Cardiology III stethoscope;

- Littman pediatric stethoscope;

- Stop watch;

- Steel measuring tape;

- Foam foot pads;

- Calibration cylinders-small, medium, large, X-large;

- Adjustable height chairs;

- Stainless steel scissors;

- Calculator;

- Pliers;

- Luer lock;

- Stethoscope eartips (small);

- Disposable pillow (17" X 23"); and

- Arm support pads.

2.3.2   Blood Pressure Supplies

- Cosmetic pencils – black (2);

- Cosmetic pencil sharpener;

- Baby oil drop dispenser bottle;

- Sani-Cloth germicidal towelettes;

- 2" x 2" gauze pads;

- Nitrile gloves;

- Masking tape;

- Mercury Spill Kit;

- Disposable pillow covers;

- Bandaids;

- Black magic marker; and

- Disposable blanket.

2.3.3   Description of Blood Pressure Equipment and Supplies

- **Baumanometer® calibrated mercury true gravity wall model sphygmomanometer.** The sphygmomanometer is factory calibrated to true gravity and is guaranteed by the manufacturer to remain scientifically accurate without need for recalibration. The mercury-gravity manometer consists of a calibrated cartridge glass tube that is optically clear, easy to clean, and abrasion resistant. The mercury reservoir at the bottom of the tube communicates with a compression cuff through a rubber tube. When air pressure is exerted on the mercury in the reservoir by pumping the pressure bulb, the mercury in the glass tube rises and indicates how much pressure the cuff applies against the artery. The manometer is connected to the wall for ease of accurate visualization. See Section 2.8 of this chapter for mercury handling procedures.

- **Baumanometer Calibrated® V-Lok® cuffs with Latex Inflation Bulb, Air-Flo Control Valve.** These cuffs come in four sizes: child, adult, large adult, and thigh. The cuffs are used with all three blood pressure instruments: mercury, aneroid, and OMRON. The Calibrated® V-Lok® compression cuff is made of urethane-coated Dacron, an unyielding material that exerts an even pressure on the inflatable bladder inside the cuff. The compression cuffs have Velcro fasteners that adhere to them to keep the cuff in position when placed on the arm. The cuff size is determined by the circumference of the arm. The size of the cuff and the bladder used influences the accuracy of the blood pressure readings—if the cuff is too narrow, the observed blood pressure is overestimated (higher than it really is), and if it is too wide, the reading may be underestimated (lower than it really is).

- **Littman™ Cardiology III stethoscope.** The stethoscopes used for listening to Korotkoff sounds are Littman™ Cardioscope III for adults and Littman™ Classic II pediatric for children. These stethoscopes are of the very highest acoustical quality. They have a bell and diaphragm chest piece, and an acoustical rating *by the manufacturer* of 9 on a scale of 1-10, with a rating of 10 having the best acoustical attributes. The construction uses a single-lumen rubber tubing connection between the ear tubes and the chest piece. The ear tubes can be adjusted to fit the particular user at an anatomically correct angle, and the plastic ear covers come in different sizes allowing the user to match the best ear canal size to achieve an acoustically sealed ear fit. All parts of the stethoscope can be cleaned for use between SPs. The bell of the stethoscope is used to auscultate the Korotkoff sounds for blood pressure measurements. Each technologist is provided with his or her own stethoscope.

- **Littman pediatric stethoscope.** A pediatric stethoscope is included for apical heart rate measurement and also can serve as an enhancement procedure for measuring blood pressure.

- **Stop watch.** The stop watch is used to measure a 60-second pulse rate during the exam.

- **Wall clock.** A 12" face clock with a second hand may be used to measure a 60-second pulse.

- **Steel measuring tape.** A retractable steel measuring tape is used to take upper arm length and circumference measurements.

- **Calibration cylinders-small, medium, large, X-large (plastic).** These cylinders are used for calibrating the sphygmomanometers and OMRON:

-	Plastic Thigh Cuff Can	20" or 51.5 cm
-	Large Arm Cuff Metal Can	13" or 33.5 cm
-	Standard Cuff Metal Can	10.5" or 26.5 cm
-	Child Cuff Metal Can	8.5" or 22 cm

- **Adjustable height chairs.** The technologists and participant are all seated during the exam. Adjustable height chairs enable positioning of the SP so that the feet rest directly on the floor, as well as assuring that the measurement technologists can adjust their seats for optimal viewing of sphygmomanometers.

- Foam Foot Pads. Foot pads are used to adjust the SP's feet so that the feet rest directly on a flat, firm surface.

- **Stainless steel scissors.** For use to cut the sleeve of the SP disposable shirt when taking blood pressure.

- **Pliers.** Pliers may be needed when changing luer locks.

- **Luer lock.** Replaces a leaking or defective luer.

- **Stethoscope eartips (small).** Replace worn eartips for the stethoscope.

- **Disposable pillow (17" X 23").** The pillow can be used to support the SP's arm when taking pulse or blood pressure.

- **Arm support pads.** Used to elevate the SP's arm to the heart level.

2.3.4   Blood Pressure Supplies – Description

- **Black cosmetic pencil.** When measuring the upper arm circumference, the technologist will make any body marks on the SP using a wax-based cosmetic pencil.

- **Baby oil drop dispenser bottle.** Baby oil is used for removing cosmetic pencil marks from the SP's skin. A small drop dispenser holds the oil for use during exams. Refills are obtained from a larger bottle of baby oil that is associated with the anthropometry component.

- **2" x 2" gauze pads.** The pads are used to wipe off cosmetic pencil marks with baby oil.

- **Sani-Cloth germicidal towelettes.** Disposable germicidal wipes are used to clean and disinfect the Dacron cuffs between participants.

- **Masking Tape.** Tape is used to pull together the cuts that were made on the SP outfit shirt when measuring the upper arm circumference.

- **Alcohol wipes.** Used to clean the steel measuring tape.

- **Mercury Spill Kit.** Used to control and clean a mercury spill.

- **Disposable pillow covers.** For use between SPs.

- **Bandaids.** Replace when the examiner must remove the bandaid that was applied during the phlebotomy.

- **Black magic marker.** Used to denote the size of BP cuff and arm circumference on the SP exam outfit shirt.

- **Wastebasket.**

2.4 HPV Supplies

- HPV Kits (150) Male and Female

    - HPV kit contents include an Epicenter tube, swab, plastic zip-closable bag, and instructions

- Dymo Costar label printer

- Dymo Costar labels

2.5 Office Supplies

The physician's room is equipped with a laser printer and is stocked with the following office supplies to support the referral process:

- Envelopes (plain and NCHS return address);

- Printer paper (plain and NCHS letterhead);

- Toner cartridge; and

- Calculator.

2.6 Emergency Supplies

- Oxygen tanks (2) Size D, 415 liters;

- Primary: Secured to wall;

- Backup: Secured to wall under desk;

- Oxygen masks and tubing (kept in tank carrying case);

- Nasal Canula: 1 adult, 1 pediatric;

- Oxygen Mask: 1 mask;

- Extension Tubing;

- Oral Airway: infant, small, medium, large; and

- Automatic External Defibrillator.

2.6.1   **Emergency Box – Contents**

- Medications

    - Albuterol Inhalers;

    - Ammonia Ampules;

    - Aspirin, 325 mg tablets;

    - Diphenhydramine liquid 12.5 mg/5ml

    - Diphenhydramine tablets 25mg

    - Epi Pen – Junior;

    - Epi Pen – Adult;

    - Glucose Tube; and

    - Nitrostat.

- Supplies

    - Protective eyewear goggles;

    - Tongue depressor;

    - Stethoscope (2) child and adult;

    - Pocket BP aneroid cuffs – child, adult, and large adult;

    - Spare AED Battery;

    - Scissors;

    - Pen light;

    - Sterile Gloves – two pairs;

- ½" Transpore tape; and

- Surgilube packets.

2.7 OSHA Bloodborne Pathogen Exposure Forms

The warehouse manager provides the forms necessary to complete the exposure evaluation reporting requirements. The bloodborne pathogen exposure protocol is found under separate cover in the *MEC Injury and Blood Exposure Procedures Manual.*

2.8 Inventory

At the beginning and end of each stand, the physician will count all component-specific equipment and supplies. Supplies ordered from the warehouse by the previous team should be on site when the next team arrives to set up a new stand. Physicians will check all newly received supplies against the associated packing lists before incorporating them into the existing inventory. After reconciling the supplies, the physician will stock the exam room. Any needed items should be noted on the inventory list, reported to the MEC manager, and documented in the Unusual Field Occurrence (UFO) system.

2.8.1 Equipment Setup

Before setting up, the physicians should verify that all equipment and supplies are in the room. Any pieces of equipment that are missing should be reported to the home office component staff who will notify NCHS staff.

All mercury manometers on the MECs are tracked in the Equipment Tracking System (ETS) maintained by the MEC manager. Provide the MEC manager with the serial numbers on each manometer at the beginning of each stand.

2.8.2 Teardown Procedure

At the end of each stand, prepare the equipment for transport as follows:

1. Pack up and secure all supplies and equipment in the cabinets and drawers. Wrap mercury manometers with bubble wrap and secure them snugly in the locked cabinet.

2. Secure the wall-mounted mercury manometer with the padded protector. The installed wall-mounted manometers do not require packing for MEC transport. See the next section for more detailed manometer handling procedures.

2.9 Handling Instructions for Mercury Manometers

2.9.1 Mercury Safety Considerations

According to the manufacturer, the elemental mercury used in Baum manometers is safely contained in the reservoir and Mylar® Clad Calibrated Cartridge glass tube. Since February 1995, Baum has applied several layers of very strong and crystal clear Mylar film to the glass tubes, which strengthen the tube and maintain its structural integrity even if the inner glass is broken. The Mylar sheath ends close to the tube's top end, and a fingernail can detect the change in the tube's outer diameter, which indicates that this tube has the Mylar film.

Handle the mercury sphygmomanometer with extreme care. The instrument should not be dropped or treated in any way that could result in damage to the manometer. Regular quality control checks are conducted to ensure that there are no leaks from the inflation system and that the manometer has not been damaged so as to cause a loss of mercury. The Baum mercury manometers are designed to minimize mercury releases from its closed system; however, there are two ways in which mercury can be released from the manometers.

One way has to do with the lever that holds the glass tube in place on top of the device only on the wall-mounted units. The lever is supposed to be moved by a service technician only when the sphygmomanometer is removed from the wall and lying on its right side. If this lever is inadvertently flipped back while the instrument is upright on the wall, the glass tube is released and the mercury spills out of the bottom of the tube. Baum has added a safety feature to this release lever: a "set screw" that prevents an accidental movement of the lever without a tool. If the unit has not been retrofitted with the set screw, a safety modification is available free of charge from Baum. The "lever lock," is simply a small piece of metal bent at a 90-degree angle that is easily slipped behind the lever to immobilize it. The lock can still be removed with no problem using a screwdriver, but spills are prevented because users cannot remove the lever lock without some effort. The lock simply eliminates the potential for anyone to accidentally flip the release lever.

The second manner in which mercury could be released is if the glass tube is damaged. With the application of Mylar® to the glass tube, the incidence of glass tube damage has been drastically reduced.

Loss of mercury will occur if the glass tube is broken in either the wall-mounted or portable manometer. Take care handling and storing the manometer to prevent this. If the tube appears cracked, check for any spilled mercury near the wall-mounted manometer.

The following procedure is recommended for handling spilled or leaking mercury:

- If you discover a mercury spill, do not attempt to clean it up yourself.

- Do not touch mercury with your bare hands or attempt to vacuum or clean up the spill.

- Leave the area in which there was a spill, taking the SP to a separate waiting area.

- Close the door to the area or room if possible.

- Obtain the Mercury Spill Kit and proceed to clean the spill.

2.9.2   **Required Procedure for Handling Spilled or Leaking Mercury**

The following procedure is required for handling spilled or leaking mercury:

- Contact the MEC manager immediately to report the incident and receive instructions. The Mercury Spill Kit contains all the materials needed for cleanup.

- The MEC manager will determine what action should be taken. If necessary, the local hazardous materials contact may be called to report such spills. The local hazardous materials agency may want to make a followup visit to the facility to check for levels of mercury in the exposed area.

- Do not touch the mercury with bare hands or attempt to vacuum or clean up the spill.

■ The procedures for cleaning up the mercury are different depending on the surface where the spill is detected.

■ If the spill is small, the following procedure may be used.

- Leakage or spillage on a hard surface (e.g., hard floor, table, etc.,):

  1. Get the Mercury Spill Kit from the physician's exam room.

  2. Put on the green protective gloves.

  3. Use the mercury (Hg Absorb) sponge.

  4. Remove the sponge from the plastic zip-closable bag.

  5. Dampen the sponge with water.

  6. Wipe the area contaminated with mercury. Do this slowly to allow for complete absorption of all free mercury. The chemical layer (Hg Absorb powder) on the sponge will absorb the mercury droplets.

  7. After finishing with the Hg Absorb sponge, place it back into its plastic zip-closable bag.

  8. Place the manometer case and mercury sponge in separate plastic bags and secure with tape. Return to the MEC manager.

  9. Complete a Mercury Spill Report Form.

  10. Obtain replacement equipment.

- Leakage and/or spillage on a soft or absorbent surface (e.g., rug, etc.):

  1. Get the Mercury Spill Kit from the physician's exam room.

  2. Put on the green protective gloves.

  3. Turn off heat or air conditioning to avoid spreading vapors to other rooms in the MEC.

  4. Open a window if possible to ensure adequate ventilation to the outside for the room where the spill occurred.

  5. Use the mercury (Hg Absorb) sponge, if possible. See directions above.

  6. Wet the MERCSORB® powder with water. Mercury will react with the powder, forming a metal/mercury amalgam.

7.   Wipe or sweep wet powder over all cracks and hard-to-reach locations for maximum pickup.

8.   Pick up amalgam by sponging or by using the small sweep and dustpan provided in the Mercury Spill Kit.

9.   Complete a Mercury Spill Report Form.

10. Obtain replacement equipment.

Follow these instructions for packing, unpacking, storing, and/or shipping a wall-mounted mercury manometer.

Wall-mounted Units

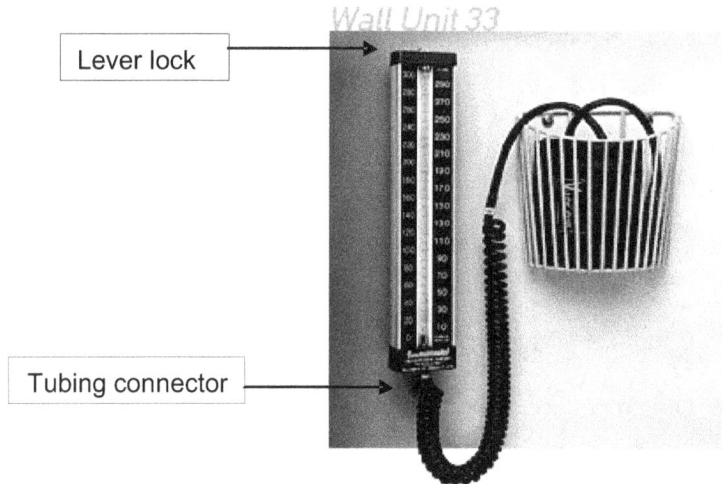

1.   Remove the coiled tubing from the instrument.

2.   Attach a red cap firmly to the tubing connector on the instrument to seal.

3.   Check that the lever lock is in place on top of instrument. If not, see attached instructions for inserting a lever lock.

4.   Remove the instrument from the wall unit.

5.   Place instrument in a zip-closable bag and seal closed.

6.   Place the instrument (in bag) in the storage box.

7.   Place storage box into zip-closable bag and seal closed.

8.   Wrap manometer box with bubble wrap.

9.   Place in storage container in physician's room for storage or, if shipping back to the warehouse, pack the manometer securely with bubble wrap in a box. The amount of mercury contained in a manometer does not require special shipping procedures in compliance with the regulations pertaining to hazardous materials.

Unpacking Manometers (wall-mounted units):

1.   Carefully inspect outer bag for mercury droplets. If no mercury is seen, open bag and remove manometer box.

2.   Open box and remove manometer. Inspect inner bag for mercury droplets. If no mercury is seen, open bag and remove manometer.

3.   Check that the lever lock or set screw is in place on top of instrument. If not, see attached instructions for inserting a lever lock.

4.   Reattach manometer to wall mount.

5.   Remove red cap from tube connector and reconnect tubing.

Lever Lock Insertion Instructions

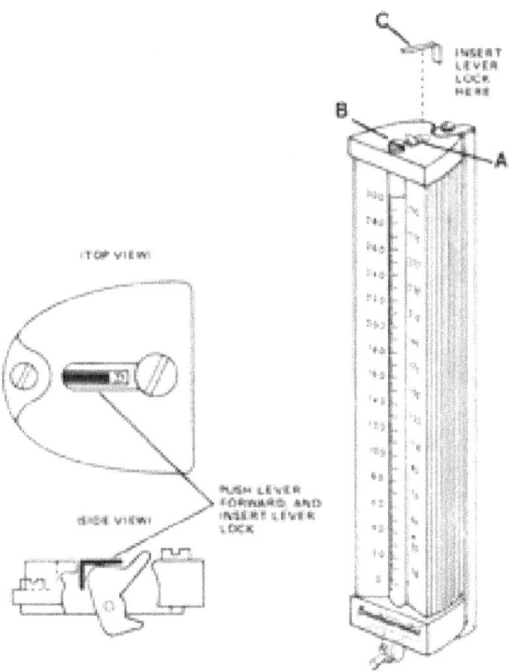

Purpose

To prevent tampering with the cartridge tube release lever and accidental release of mercury.

Procedure

Push lever "A" forward (toward the chrome plated cap "B") and insert lever lock "C" as shown in diagram.

Desk-top Models

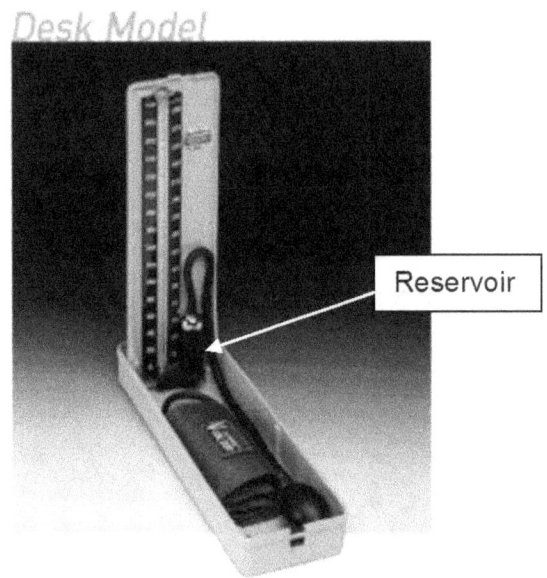

Packing desk-top manometers:

1. Remove tubing from top of reservoir.

2. Tilt manometer onto reservoir-side. Mercury should be contained in reservoir.

3. Place red cap firmly on reservoir opening while manometer is on its side.

4. Stand manometer up. Close.

5. Place manometer in zip-closable bag and seal closed.

6. Place manometer (in bag) in storage box.

7. Place storage box in zip-closable bag and seal closed.

8. Wrap manometer box with bubble wrap.

9. Place in storage container in physician's room for transport to next stand.

Unpacking Manometers (Desk-top model):

1. Carefully inspect outer bag for mercury droplets. If no mercury is seen, open bag and remove manometer box.

2. Open box and remove manometer. Inspect inner bag for mercury droplets. If no mercury is seen, open bag and remove manometer.

3. Open manometer and place upright on table.

4. Remove red cap from reservoir and reconnect tubing.

3. PHYSICIAN PROTOCOL

General Overview

This chapter presents the physician examination protocol only. The other roles the physician fills are presented in Chapters 5 and 6.

The physician protocol includes the following:

- 3.1. Heart Rate, Pulse, and Blood Pressure Measurements;

- 3.2. Blood Pressure Measurement Screens;

- 3.3. Shared Exclusion Questions; and

- 3.4. Sexually Transmitted Diseases (STD) and Human Immunodeficiency Virus (HIV) Testing .

3.1 Heart Rate, Pulse, and Blood Pressure Measurements

Physicians fill a central role on the mobile examination center (MEC) team with the primary functions of collecting blood pressure and heart rate/pulse data. Apical heart rates are measured on all children up to and including 4 years of age. Radial (brachial if necessary) pulses are measured on SPs aged 5 years and older. Blood pressures and radial pulses are measured on all SPs aged 8 years and older.

Age	Measurements
0 – 4	Apical heart rate
5 – 8	Radial pulse
8 +	Radial pulse and blood pressure

The protocol for blood pressure measurement follows procedures developed by the American Heart Association. Physicians and backup physicians are certified in blood pressure measurement through a training program provided by SHARED Care Inc., that includes didactic information, video practice, listening to and recording Korotkoff sounds, and practice listening to blood pressures of volunteers with a certified instructor. Certification is achieved when physicians meet all requirements of the training program. Recertification is accomplished quarterly.

3.1.1 Procedures for Heart Rate, Pulse, and Blood Pressure Measurements

3.1.2 Heart Rate Measurements for SPs through Age 4

For all SPs through the age of 4 years, only the apical heart rate is recorded. Count the heart rate by listening to the heart at approximately the 4th intercostal space, midclavicular line. Use the bell device of the pediatric stethoscope.

- Remove all clothing over the left chest wall.

- The heart rate should be recorded after the child rests for 4 minutes.

- If the SP is extremely active or crying, allow an additional maximum of 2 minutes for him or her to become quiet before counting the heart rate.

- If the child can sit in a chair without an adult, have the child sit quietly in the chair until the heart rate is counted.

- If the child needs to be held, ask the adult who accompanies the child to hold the child in an upright position without "squeezing" any portion of the body, especially the abdomen.

- Count the rate for 30 seconds and record it in the ISIS **Heart Rate Field**.

- Note regularity and record in the ISIS **Regular Field**.

3.1.2.1 Pulse Measurements for All SPs Ages 5 and older

For all SPs aged 5 years and older, a palpated radial pulse rate is recorded.

- The pulse may be taken after the SP has been seated and resting quietly for approximately 4 minutes.

- With the elbow and forearm resting comfortably on a table and the palm of the hand turned upward, find the radial pulse and count for 30 seconds.

- The number of beats in 30 seconds is recorded.

- The **rhythm field** is defaulted to "Regular." If there is an irregular rhythm, click on the radio button indicating regular, and check the box to specify "Irregular."

  - If the SP is between ages 6 and 79, the system will enable a space to enter the number of irregular beats that occurred in 60 seconds.

- Count the pulse again for 60 seconds and record the number of missed beats during that period. Enter this number in the appropriate box. If there are four or more missed beats in 60 seconds, the system will block the SP from the bronchodilator component.

3.1.2.2 Procedures for Measuring Blood Pressures and Pulse for Participants Aged 8 Years and Older

For the purpose of standardization, both pulse and blood pressure are measured in the right arm unless specific SP conditions prohibit the use of the right arm, or if SPs self-report any reason that the blood pressure procedure should not be taken in the right arm. If the measurements cannot be taken in the right arm, they are taken in the left arm. In all cases, if there is a problem with both arms, the blood pressure is not taken. There are no protocol-specific reasons for excluding SPs from pulse measurement.

3.1.2.3 SPs Excluded from Blood Pressure

SPs are excluded from blood pressure measurement if they have any condition that could potentially cause them harm or discomfort or that would prevent accurate blood pressure measurement. BP measurements are not done when both arms have a rash, gauze/adhesive dressings, casts, are withered, puffy, have tubes, open sores, hematomas, wounds, arteriovenous (AV) shunt, or any other intravenous access device. Also, women who have had an axillary nodal biopsy or resection or a unilateral radical mastectomy do not have their blood pressure measured in the affected arm. If there is a condition with both arms, the blood pressure is not taken.

3.1.3 Blood Pressure Premeasurement Procedure

Several steps must be followed before taking the first blood pressure. This section presents these steps, also referred to as blood pressure premeasurement procedures. They are:

- Open physician application by scanning the SP ID bracelet;

- If necessary, measure arm circumference;

- Seat participant in the chair and position for blood pressure;

- Explain procedure;

- Identify brachial and upper arm pulses;

- Apply blood pressure cuff; and

- Start a 5-minute rest period.

3.1.3.1   Open the Physician Application

As soon as the SP arrives, the SP ID bracelet must be scanned to launch the physician application.

3.1.3.2   Arm Circumference Protocol to Determine Cuff Size

In the anthropometry exam, the right upper arm circumference is measured; if the SP has not yet been to the body measures component, the physician will measure the upper arm circumference. This is solely to determine the blood pressure cuff size; the SP will have the formal survey arm circumference measured again in the anthropometry component.

First, measure the length of upper arm:

- **Position the SP:** Direct the SP to turn away from you. Ask him or her to stand upright with the weight evenly distributed on both feet, the right arm bent 90° at the elbow, and the right palm facing up. Demonstrate the correct position if necessary.

- **Mark the measurement site:** Locate the end of the spine of the right scapula by following the scapula out to the arm until it makes a sharp V-turn to the front of the body (Exhibit 3-1). Using the cosmetic pencil, make a horizontal line on the **uppermost edge of the posterior border** of the scapula spine extending from the acromion process (see Exhibit 3-2).

- **Take the measurement:** Hold the zero end of the measuring tape at this mark and extend the tape down the **center** of the posterior surface of the arm to the tip of the olecranon process, the bony part of the mid-elbow (Exhibit 3-3). Take the measurement to the nearest 0.1 cm.

- **Mark the midpoint:** Divide the value in half to calculate the midpoint of the measured length. Holding the tape in place, make a horizontal mark at the midpoint and cross this mark with a **perpendicular line centered** on the posterior surface of the arm (see Exhibit 3-5). This mark defines the site at which the arm circumference will be measured. Tell the SP to then relax the right arm and let it hang loosely

- Next, measure arm circumference:

■ **Position the SP:** Ask the SP to turn so that you stand **facing** his or her right side. Do not stand behind the SP for this measurement. Have the participant stand upright with the weight evenly distributed on both feet, the shoulders relaxed, and the right arm hanging loosely at the sides. Flexing or tightening the arm muscles will yield an inaccurate measurement.

■ **Take the measurement:** Wrap the measuring tape around the arm at the level of the upper arm mid-point mark. Position the tape **perpendicular** to the long axis of the upper arm. Pull the two ends of the overlapping tape together so that the zero end sits below the measurement value and the result lies on the lateral aspect of the arm (not the posterior surface). Check that the tape fits snugly around the arm but does not compress the skin (Exhibit 3-3).

Exhibit 3-1. Upper arm bony landmarks

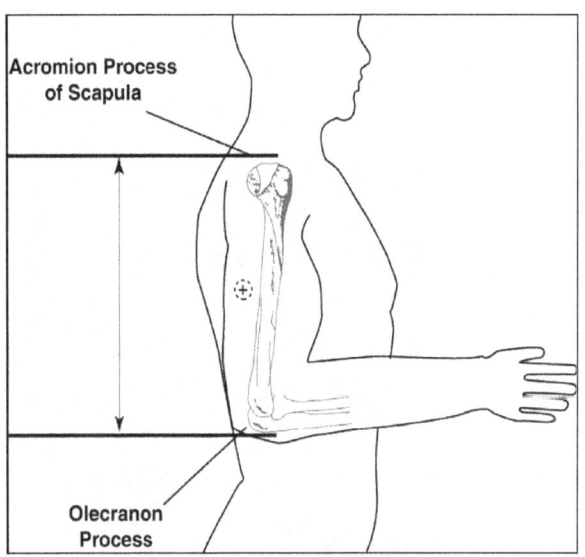 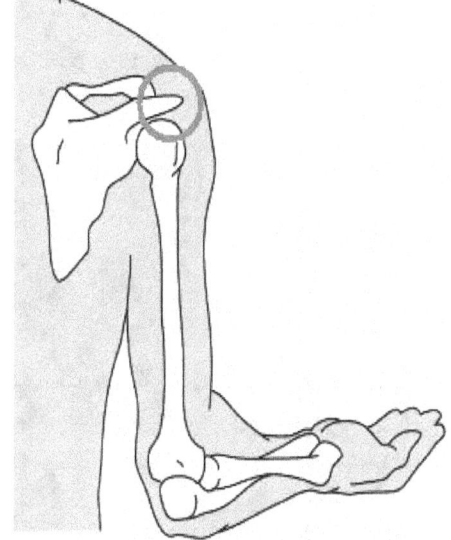

Exhibit 3-2. Marking spine extending
from acromion process

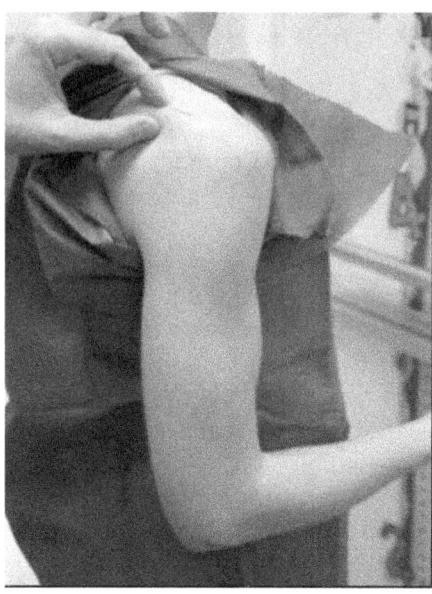

Exhibit 3-3. **CORRECT** tape placement
for upper arm length

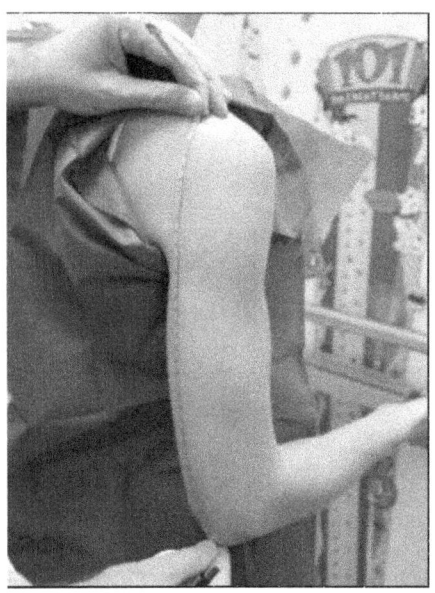

Exhibit 3-4. **INCORRECT** tape placement
for upper arm length

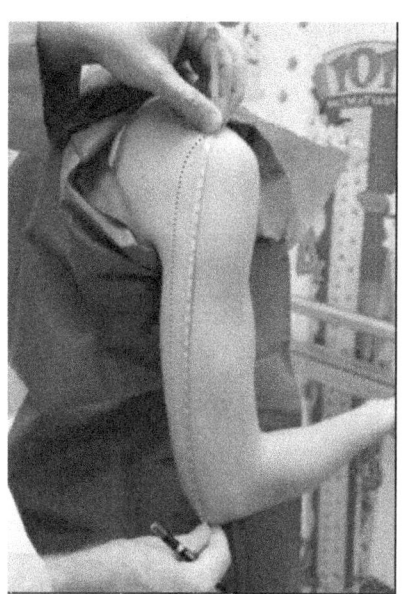

IMPORTANT: The tape must be centered on the posterior surface of the arm. Exhibit 3-3 shows the
correct placement of the measuring tape centered on the posterior surface of the arm; Exhibit 3-4 shows
the measuring tape placed incorrectly.

Exhibit 3-5. Marking upper arm length midpoint

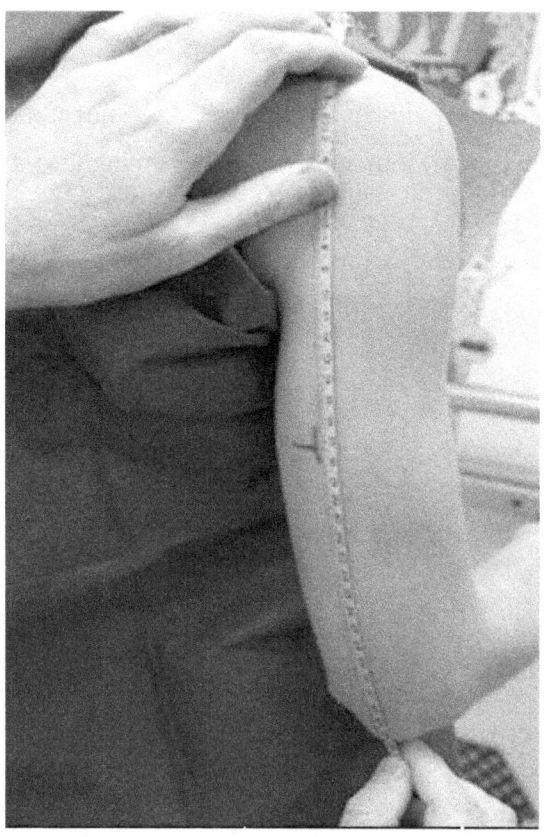

3.1.3.3   Position SP for Pulse and Blood Pressure Measurements

The SP sits in a height-adjustable office style chair. Ask the SP to sit all the way to the back of the chair so that the spine is straight. The back should be supported and both feet should rest flat on the floor, and the SP should appear comfortable. Shorter SPs may need the chair height lowered; tall SPs may need the chair height raised to correctly position for the BP measurement. If necessary, place SP's feet on a foot stool or floor pads.

The arm should be bared and unrestricted by clothing. Position the arm on the table with the palm of the hand turned upward and the elbow slightly flexed. The midpoint of the upper arm should be at the level of the heart, located at the junction of the fourth intercostal space. Very tall SPs may need to place their arm on an arm rest or pillow to bring their upper arm to the correct position.

3.1.3.4   Explain the Procedure

Inform the SP that you will be taking a series of three and perhaps four blood pressure measurements. The talking points below can assist you in describing the protocol.

"I am going to take a series of three different blood pressures. Before taking your first blood pressure reading there will be a 5-minute waiting period.

In order for us to take accurate blood pressure readings, it is important that, during the waiting period, and during the blood pressure measurements, you:

- Sit up straight with your back against the back of the chair, making sure to keep both feet flat on the floor.

- Because moving and talking can change your blood pressure, we ask you not to talk or move your position while I am taking your blood pressure.

- After the resting period, I will take your pulse and then I will take three or four blood pressure readings.

- Do you have any questions?"

Stress the quiet period as a very important part of the blood pressure protocol. Also, the examiner must observe the SP's position throughout the blood pressure protocol because of the natural tendency for people to want to cross their feet or legs.

Inform the SP that, before taking the first blood pressure, you will take the pulse and then determine how high to inflate the cuff by taking the pulse while inflating the cuff.

3.1.3.5   Locate Brachial Pulses

Two brachial pulses are palpated and marked: the upper arm and antecubital brachial pulses.

Upper Arm Brachial Pulse

The purpose of palpating and marking this pulse is for the proper application of the blood pressure cuff.

Position the SP with the right palm turned upward and the arm slightly bent at the elbow. Palpate the brachial pulse in the groove between the bicep and tricep muscles above the elbow with the pads of the index and middle fingers. Using an eyeliner pencil, mark the spot where the pulse is most strongly palpated. **The center of the cuff bladder will be placed at this point.**

Antecubital Brachial Pulse

The purpose of palpating and marking this pulse is to locate the strongest pulse landmark for the consistent placement of the stethoscope for each blood pressure.

Trace the brachial pulse from the bicep and tricep space until palpated in the medial aspect of the antecubital fossa. Mark the spot using the eyeliner pencil. This is the point where the bell of the stethoscope is placed to listen for the BP.

If you cannot feel the pulse in the arm, check the radial pulse. If no radial or brachial pulse is palpable on the right arm, use the left arm unless contraindicated. If a radial pulse is apparent, whether or not the brachial pulse can be felt, attempt the blood pressure measurement.

3.1.3.6   Apply Blood Pressure Cuff

Using Table 3-1, locate the arm circumference and corresponding cuff size.

Table 3-1. Arm circumference and corresponding cuff size

Cuff size	Bladder width (cm)	Bladder length (cm)	Arm circumference[1]
Child	9	17	17-21.9
Adult	12	22	22-29.9
Large adult	15	32	30-37.9
Adult thigh	18	35	38-47.9

[1]Pickering, T.G., et al. Recommendations for Blood Pressure Measurements in Humans and Experimental Animals. Part 1: Blood Pressure in Humans. *Hypertension* 2005, 45: 142-161. Originally published online December 20, 2004.

Blood Pressure Cuff Size and Application

Measure the arm circumference to determine the accurate cuff bladder size. The length and width of the cuff's bladder should encircle at least 80 percent of the length of the arm and 40 percent of the width of an adult's arm. In children under 13 years, the length and width of the bladder should encircle 100 percent of the arm. The index lines on the BP cuffs are not used to guide cuff application in this study.

- Use the cuff size from column 1 associated with the arm circumference in column 4. (Example: If the arm circumference at midpoint is 36 cm, use the large adult cuff.)

- Position the center of the *rubber bladder* over the upper arm brachial artery mark at least **1" *above the crease of the elbow.*** For long thin arms, place the cuff in the middle of the arm. Place the marker on the inner part of the cuff directly over the brachial artery.

- Wrap the cuff in a circular manner taking care not to wrap it in a spiral direction.

- Check the fit of the cuff to ensure that it is secure but not tight. Two fingers should fit under the cuff.

Some upper arm physiques can present special challenges in the proper application of a cuff. For example, a very short upper arm with a large circumference that tapers markedly toward the antecubital space presents a special challenge. In this case, the cuff may be wrapped in a spiraling direction rather than keeping the edges even around the arm. Also, applying the thigh cuff to an upper arm can be bulky and awkward. In all cases, the objective is to achieve the best contact of the bladder with the cuff so that the bladder inflates in the proper position over the brachial artery.

The 5-Minute Rest Period

Inform the SP that the 5-minute rest period will begin, and again reinforce that no conversing will take place from that point on until the end of the blood pressure measurements. The Blood Pressure Pre-measurement ISIS application screen contains a radio button that begins the 5-minute timer when clicked. During this rest period, the physician often finds it a good time to review the referral screen. The formal rest period lasts 3 minutes. You may quietly coach the SP to maintain his or her position seated with feet flat on the floor, looking straight ahead. The SP must rest for a full 3 minutes. After 3 minutes, you can measure the pulse; at 4 minutes, the maximum inflation level can be obtained. During the rest period, because of the natural tendency for people to want to cross their feet or legs, continually observe the SP's position.

Radial Pulse Measurement

Take the pulse after the SP has been seated and resting quietly for at least 3 minutes. Position the arm with the right palm upward. Palpate the radial pulse on the lateral flexor surface of the wrist with the pads of the index and middle fingers. Count the pulse for 30 seconds and enter the number of beats in a 30-second period in the heart rate field. The physician can use a digital stopwatch or a wall clock with a second hand to time the pulse measurement. The system calculates this rate and displays the number of beats in 60 seconds on the screen. Next, note whether the rhythm is irregular and estimate the number of missed beats.

3.1.3.7   Determine the Maximum Inflation Level (MIL)

The maximum inflation level (MIL) is measured after the SP has been seated and resting quietly for **at least 4 minutes**. The examiner must calculate and document the MIL in the application before taking the first blood pressure reading. The MIL or palpatory method provides an approximation of the systolic blood pressure and represents the highest level to which the cuff should be inflated before taking the first blood pressures. The primary objective of measuring the MIL is to assure that the cuff is inflated above a possible auscultatory gap.

The auscultatory gap is a normal blood pressure variation in which at least two repetitive Korotkoff sounds are followed by a temporary absence of sound, or a gap. This gap may last for a few mm Hg or as long as 40 mm Hg. The failure to compensate for a possible auscultatory gap increases the likelihood of two distinct measurement errors: (1) missing the true systolic by failing to inflate to a point above the true systolic, resulting in a falsely low systolic measurement and (2) failing to listen long enough, thus missing the end of the gap which results in a falsely high diastolic measurement.

The MIL is determined as follows:

- The mercury manometer should be positioned at eye level so the mercury meniscus can be easily read without parallax.

- Locate the radial pulse in the right arm;

- While palpating the radial pulse, inflate the cuff quickly to a pressure of 70 – 80 mm Hg;

- Inflate the cuff in increments of 10 mm Hg until the radial pulse is no longer palpable (palpated systolic);

- Continue inflating the cuff in increments of 10 mm Hg to a final measure that is 30 mm Hg above the pressure where the pulse was last palpated. This number is the MIL. Note this measurement and record in the application;

- Rapidly deflate the cuff, confirm the return of the pulse, and disconnect the tubing between the cuff and the manometer; and

- If you cannot obtain the MIL on the first attempt, wait 1 minute and repeat the process. Enter the MIL in the **MIL Field** in the Premeasurement Screen.

3.1.3.8   Mercury Manometer Blood Pressure Readings

Blood pressure readings may begin after the SP has been seated and resting quietly for **at least 5 minutes**. Three consecutive blood pressure readings are obtained, using the same arm. If a blood the examiner cannot hear one or more of the readings (systolic or diastolic), a fourth attempt may be made. The increments of the mercury manometer markings are in 2-mm intervals. All end digit BP measurements should be recorded as even numbered digits.

The procedure follows:

- Place earpieces of the stethoscope into the ear canals;

- Confirm that the stethoscope head is in the low-frequency (bell) position. The bell is recommended because it may be better suited to hear the low frequency sounds;

- Position the bell of the stethoscope over the brachial artery marking and hold it firmly in place, making sure that the head makes contact with the skin around its entire circumference. If possible, avoid allowing the cuff, tubing, or bell to come in contact with each other;

- Rapidly and steadily inflate the cuff to the MIL;

- When the MIL is reached, open the thumb valve and smoothly deflate the cuff at a constant rate near 2-mm Hg per second (one mark or dial tick per second) while listening for systolic and diastolic blood pressure sounds;

- Keep the center of the manometer at eye level;

- Watch the top of the mercury column (meniscus) as the pressure in the bladder falls and note points at which the first repetitive sounds are heard (Phase I) and when they disappear (Phase V);

- Continue steady deflation at 2 mm Hg per second for at least another 10 mm Hg past where the last sounds were heard;

- Rapidly deflate the cuff and disconnect the manometer tubing from the inflation cuff between measurements to ensure that it deflates completely to zero (begin 30- second count);

- Wait 30 seconds between readings with the SP resting quietly, making sure that he or she maintains the proper position;

- While waiting for the 30-second count between measurements, record Phase I (the level of the pressure on the manometer at the first appearance of repetitive sounds) as the systolic blood pressure reading;

- Record Phase V (the point at which the last muffled sound is heard) as the diastolic blood pressure reading;

- If Phase I or Phase V occurs between the millimeter marks on the glass column, round **upward** to the nearest digit;

- Take a second set of measurements and record the systolic and diastolic pressures in the system;

- Disconnect the manometer tubing and wait 30 seconds between readings with the SP resting quietly; and

- Take the third measurement and record the systolic and diastolic pressures in the system.

When all of the measurements are complete, remove cuff and wipe all cosmetic pencil markings using baby oil and 2"x 2" gauze pads.

The following "Mercury Blood Pressure Measurement Protocol Checklist" is available on all MECs as a guide.

Table 3-2. Mercury Blood Pressure Measurement Protocol Checklist

Mercury Blood Pressure Measurement Protocol Checklist
Premeasurement Procedures:
Scan SPID barcode to launch the physician application when SP enters the room.
Measure arm circumference if needed before SP is seated.
Seat SP in the chair and position for BP.
Explain procedure and the desired examination environment.
Palpate/mark brachial arterial pulse in upper arm.
Palpate/mark brachial arterial pulse.
Select cuff size, apply cuff, and test fit.
Inform the SP that the quiet period will now begin, and press the "Timer Start" button.
Continually observe SP's position and correct if necessary during resting period and blood pressure measurements.

At 3 Minutes	Obtain radial pulse minutes and note rhythm.
At 4 Minutes	Connect manometer tubing to cuff tubing and measure MIL.
At 5 Minutes	Begin 3 blood pressure measurements.

Confirm correct stethoscope placement over brachial artery.
Observe the correct inflation and deflation rates.
Use enhancements if the first reading is difficult to hear.
Disconnect the manometer tubing between readings.
Wait 30 seconds between readings.
Take a 4th blood pressure if any CNOs were obtained.
Remove cuff.
Remove marks on SP's arm with baby oil, and tape the SP's shirt sleeve together.
Discuss results with the SP.

3.1.4　　Additional Blood Pressure Measurement Guidelines

The examiner will often encounter issues for which some guidelines exist. The following points will address the most commonly encountered blood pressure problems.

Maximum Number of Cuff Inflations

The maximum number of cuff inflations for each SP in the mercury measurement is **five,** counting all MIL attempts and blood pressure attempts. The rationale for this is twofold: to minimize the discomfort to the SP of frequent cuff inflations and to accomplish data collection for this measurement within the time allowed.

Faint Korotkoff Sounds

If the blood pressure sounds are not heard during the first measurement, indicate "Could Not Obtain" (CNO) in the computer application. It is not possible to document a systolic or diastolic reading accompanied by a CNO. The entire reading is invalid. Every time a CNO is obtained, you first assure that the stethoscope position was directly over the brachial pulse and check the BP tubing for loose connections or tubing kinks.

If there are no instrument issues, you must use an enhancement method when taking the next blood pressure. Do not attempt another measurement hoping the sounds will improve without an enhancement.

Two methods can be used to increase the intensity and volume of the sounds:

- Consider using the pediatric bell stethoscope. The reduced surface area of the pediatric sized bell can improve the volume of Korotkoff sounds.

- Inflate the cuff, then have the SP open and close his or her fist several times (6 to 8 times). Blood pressure is then determined in the usual manner. The physician inventory includes a rubber squeeze ball to help the SP squeeze his or her hand.

A third, but rarely used enhancement is available but is advised only if the first two enhancements fail to improve Korotkoff sounds. In this enhancement, the examiner elevates the SP's arm above the level of the heart before and during inflation, and then lowers the arm after the cuff has been inflated to the MIL. This method can be awkward because the movement of the arm can affect the position of the stethoscope over the brachial artery.

When an enhancement method is used to measure blood pressures (BP), check **"enhancement" field** on the data entry screen for that measurement.

First Systolic Reading Falls Within 10 mm HG of the MIL

In a small percentage of MIL calculations, the first systolic blood pressure is measured within 10 mm Hg; for example, the MIL is palpated at 130 and the first systolic blood pressure measurement is 126. The blood pressure application features a hard edit when the first systolic blood pressure is 9 mm or less than the MIL. The application will not accept the systolic reading and the reading should be entered as "CNO (Could Not Obtain). Given that it is preferable to use the available remaining inflations to obtain blood pressure readings rather than recalculating the MIL, it is not necessary to repalpate the MIL.

- Document "CNO" for the first BP measurement. That will prompt the application to automatically display a field for a 4th blood pressure reading.

- Return to the premeasurement screen (first BP screen) and change the MIL to reflect your first systolic blood pressure + 30.

- Advance to the second blood pressure measurement screen and continue.

- Take a 4th blood pressure if the SP is tolerating the procedure.

3.1.4.1   Hard Edit Limits for Blood Pressure

A hard edit is a limit imposed by the system that prevents data entry above or below the specified instrument or measurable limits. When entries are recorded that are outside these limits, the system displays a message that the value is out of range and sends a "pop-up message" asking that the value be reentered. The system will not allow entries that are outside the specified hard edit limits. The hard edits imposed by the system are listed below:

- Systolic blood pressure and maximum inflation level cannot be greater than 300 mm Hg. This is the upper range of the measurement device. The mercury manometer has a minimum and maximum scale of 0 to 300, respectively. It is impossible to get a reading above or below this level.

- Systolic and diastolic blood pressure and maximum inflation level can be even numbers only. This is a function of the measurement device. The manometer displays the readings in increments of 2.

- Systolic blood pressure must be greater than diastolic blood pressure.

- If there is no systolic blood pressure, there can be no diastolic blood pressure. (However, there can be a systolic measurement without a diastolic measurement.)

- Systolic blood pressure cannot be zero (diastolic blood pressure can be zero).

3.1.4.2   Soft Edit Limits for Blood Pressure

A soft edit is a limit imposed by the system if a value is outside the predefined edit limits for the SP being measured. The predefined edits are based on NHANES III data. When measures outside these values are recorded, the system displays a pop-up message warning that the limit is out of range, and asks if the measurement is correct. The person entering the data has the option of editing or accepting that data value. Soft edits are placed on heart rate, pulse, and systolic and diastolic blood pressures. The soft edits applied by the system are listed below.

- The difference between systolic BP and diastolic BP cannot be less than 20 mm Hg or greater than 100 mm Hg.

- Maximum inflation level should be greater than systolic blood pressure.

- Systolic BP minimum and maximum ages 8-19—76 to 130 mm Hg

- Diastolic BP minimum and maximum ages 8-19—20 to 85 mm Hg

- Systolic BP minimum and maximum ages 20-49—86 to 160 mm Hg

- Diastolic BP minimum and maximum ages 20-49—50 to 100 mm Hg

- Systolic BP minimum and maximum ages 50+—90 to 200 mm Hg

- Diastolic BP minimum and maximum ages 50+—50 to 106 mm Hg

- Pulse minimum and maximum all ages, males and females 40 to 190 beats/minute

3.1.4.3   Averaging Rules for Determining Mean Blood Pressure

- The physician application calculates the blood pressure average using the following protocol:

  - If only one blood pressure reading was obtained, that reading is the average.

  - If there is more than one blood pressure reading, the first reading is always excluded from the average.

  - If two blood pressure readings were obtained, the second blood pressure reading is the average.

  - If all diastolic readings were zero, then the average would be zero.

- Exception: If there is one diastolic reading of zero and one (or more) with a number above zero, the diastolic reading with zero is not used to calculate the diastolic average.

  - If two out of three are zero, the one diastolic reading that is not zero is used to calculate the diastolic average.

3.1.5   Data Entry Screens for Pulse and Blood Pressure

The following sections instruct physicians about how to carry out the data entry for the physician component. The ISIS screens are displayed as a visual reference.

3.1.5.1   Child Heart Rate, Pulse

Heart rate (0-4 years of age) or pulse (5-7 years of age) is counted for 30 seconds and the number of beats in a 30-second period is entered in the heart rate field. The system calculates this rate and displays the number of beats in 60 seconds on the screen. The 60-second heart rates are stored in the database (Exhibit 3-6).

Exhibit 3-6. Child heart rate/pulse

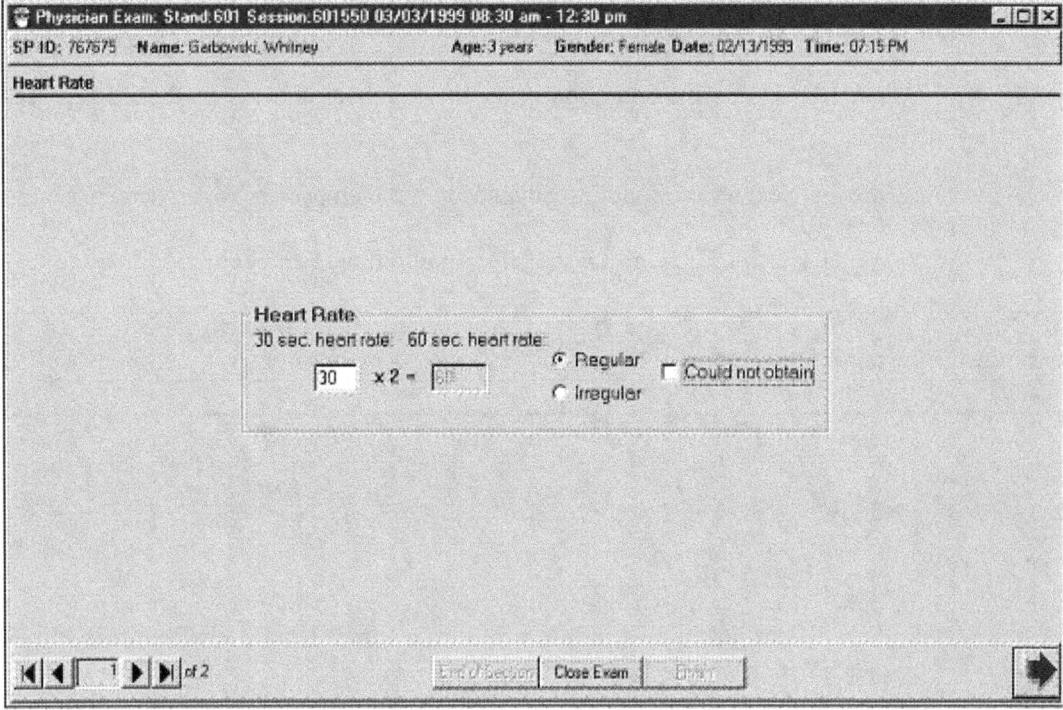

- Enter the 30-second heart rate or pulse in the field. The system calculates the 60-second heart rate and displays it in the **60-second heart rate field.**

- When taking the heart rate and pulse, note whether it is regular or irregular. The default is regular. If the heart rate is irregular, click the **irregular field option** box.

- If the next button is pressed before the heart rate is entered, a message is displayed: "Please enter heart rate or check Could not Obtain." (Exhibit 3-7).

- Click OK to this message and enter the number of beats in the **30-sec. heart rate** field.

- Click the Next arrow button to advance to the Component Status screen.

Exhibit 3-7. Child heart rate: Required data entry

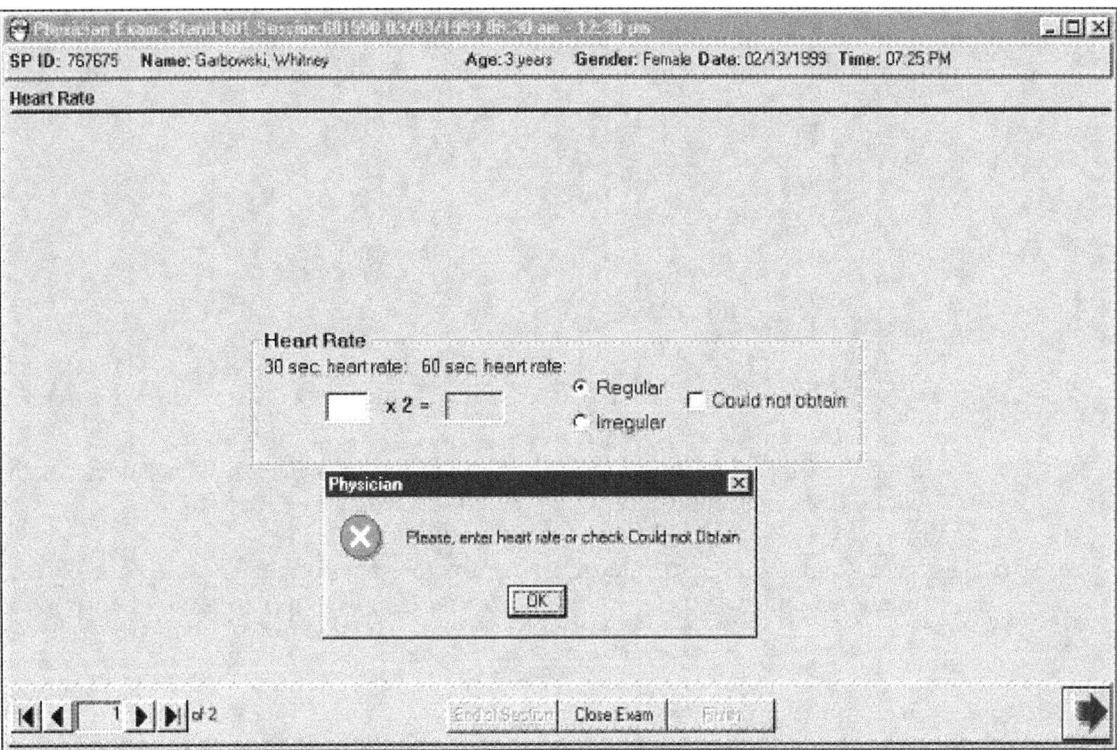

- If the heart rate was entered, the component status defaults to "complete."

- If the heart rate was not done, the status defaults to "partial."

- Select an appropriate comment from the drop-down list.

- Select the Finish button to close the examination. (Exhibit 3-8).

Exhibit 3-8. Component status for child heart rate/pulse

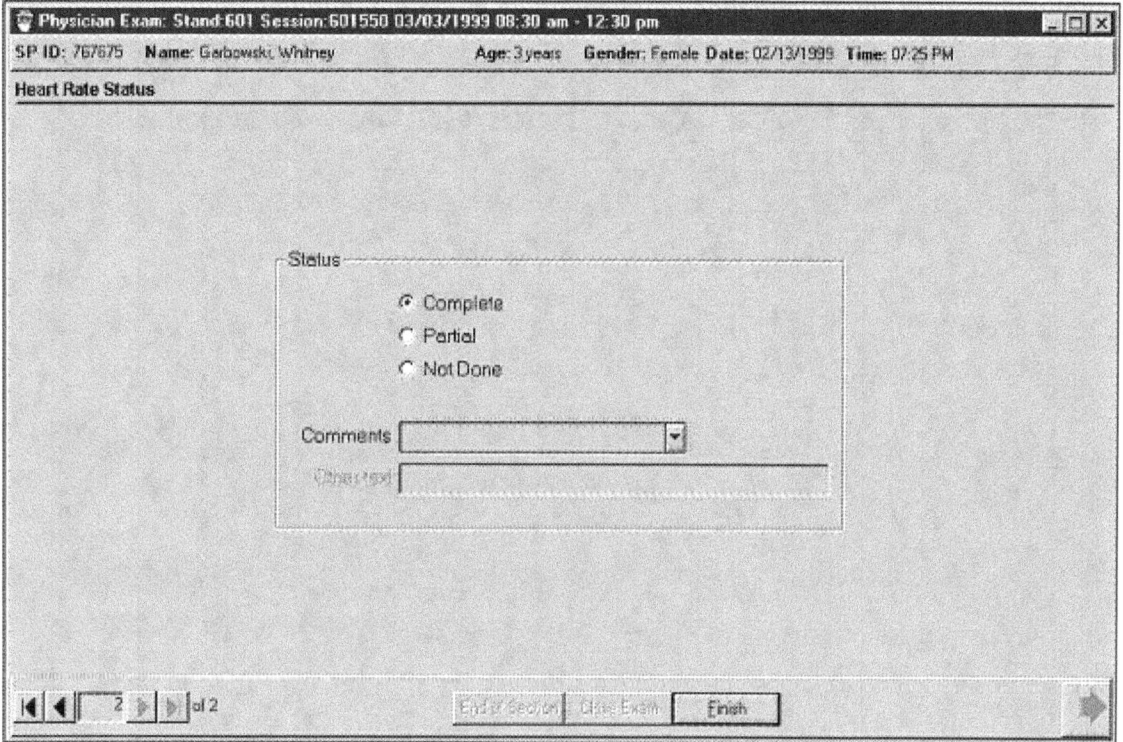

3.1.5.2 Blood Pressure Data Entry

- Ask if the SP has had food, alcohol, coffee, or cigarettes in the last 30 minutes. Check all that apply. Answering "Yes" does not exclude SPs from any of the physician's examination.

- A timer on the right side of the screen starts a 5-minute count when this screen is opened. The timer is used to help determine when the pulse, MIL, and blood pressure measurements are to be made (Exhibit 3-9).

Exhibit 3-9. Default blood pressure screen

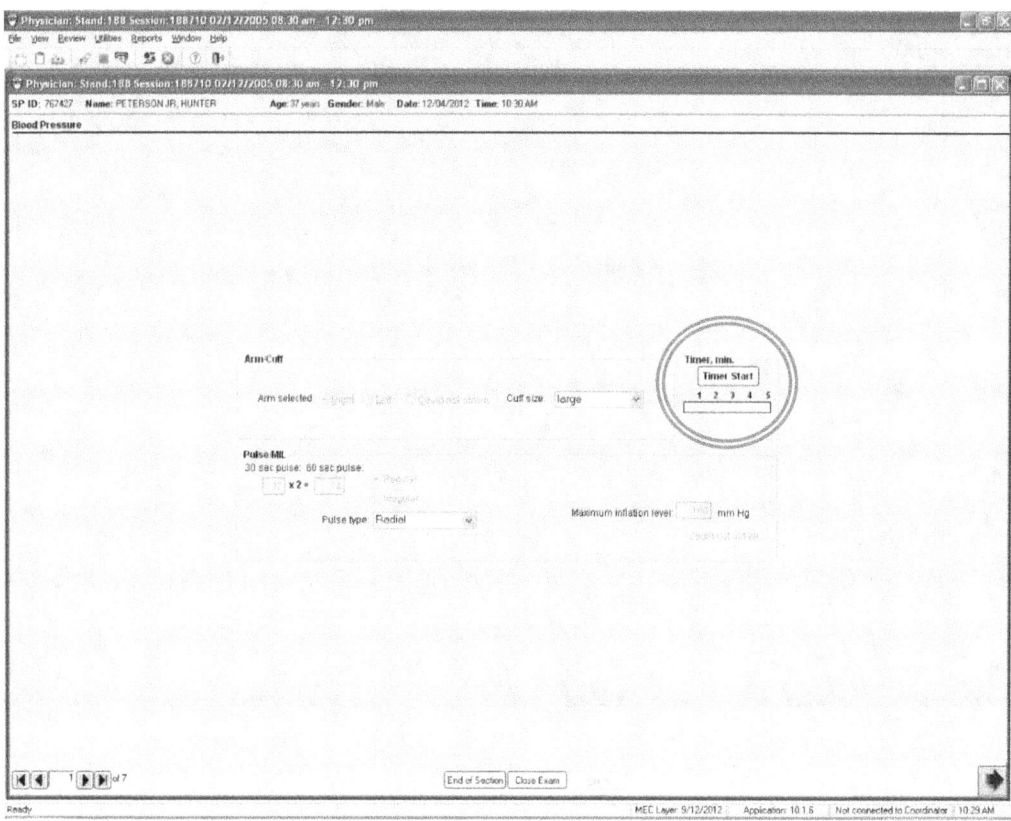

- The pulse should not be taken until the SP has been resting quietly for **at least** 3 minutes. The SP should be seated quietly during this time to allow the heart rate and blood pressure measurements to stabilize to a standard resting state.

- The MIL should not be taken until the SP has been resting quietly for **at least** 4 minutes.

- The blood pressure should not be taken until the SP has been resting for **at least** 5 minutes.

- The default for "Arm/cuff" is the right arm. If the left arm is used, click on left.

- If "Could not Obtain" is selected, the cuff size, MIL, and blood pressure fields are disabled.

- Check which arm is being used for the BP. The system defaults to the right arm.

- Select the BP cuff size from the drop-down menu. The sizes of cuffs are child, adult, large adult, and adult thigh (Exhibit 3-10).

Exhibit 3-10. Blood pressure cuff size

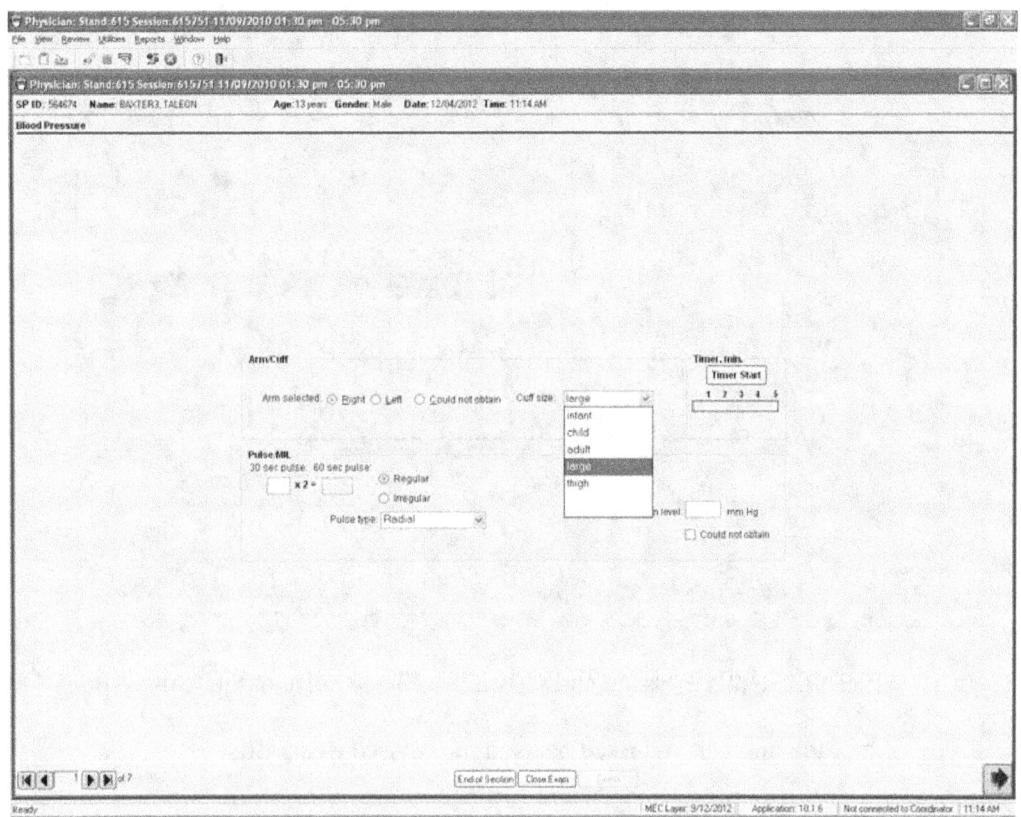

- If the cuff size is not selected before the Next button is pressed, a message is displayed with a reminder to select cuff size.

- The default site for taking the pulse is radial. If the radial pulse is not palpable, try the brachial. If a brachial pulse is obtained, select and record brachial from the drop-down menu of the "Pulse Type" field.

- Enter the 30-second pulse in the "30-sec pulse" field. The system will automatically calculate the 60-second heart rate and display it on the screen.

- Note whether the heart rate was regular or irregular. If the heart rate was irregular, click the box indicating irregular.

- The default pulse type is radial. If the pulse type was brachial, use the drop-down menu to change the pulse type to brachial.

- If the physician tries to exit from this screen before recording the pulse measurement, a system message is displayed: "Please, enter Pulse or check Could not Obtain." (Exhibit 3-11).

Exhibit 3-11. Required pulse entry

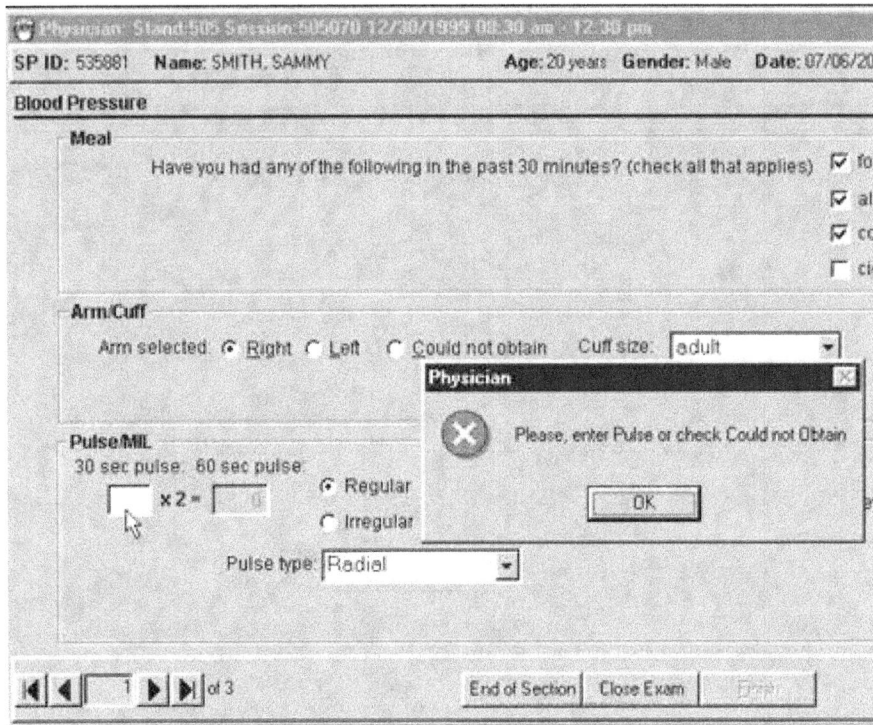

- Click OK to this message and record the 30-sec pulse in the "30-sec pulse" field.

- Enter the number of missed beats in the Missed Beats Box.

■ Get the maximum inflation level (MIL) and enter this in the "Maximum inflation level" data entry field. If a number greater than 300 is entered a message is displayed: "The value you entered is out of range. Please reenter your reading." The mercury manometer does not register numbers greater than 300 (Exhibit 3-12).

Exhibit 3-12. Out-of-range maximum inflation level

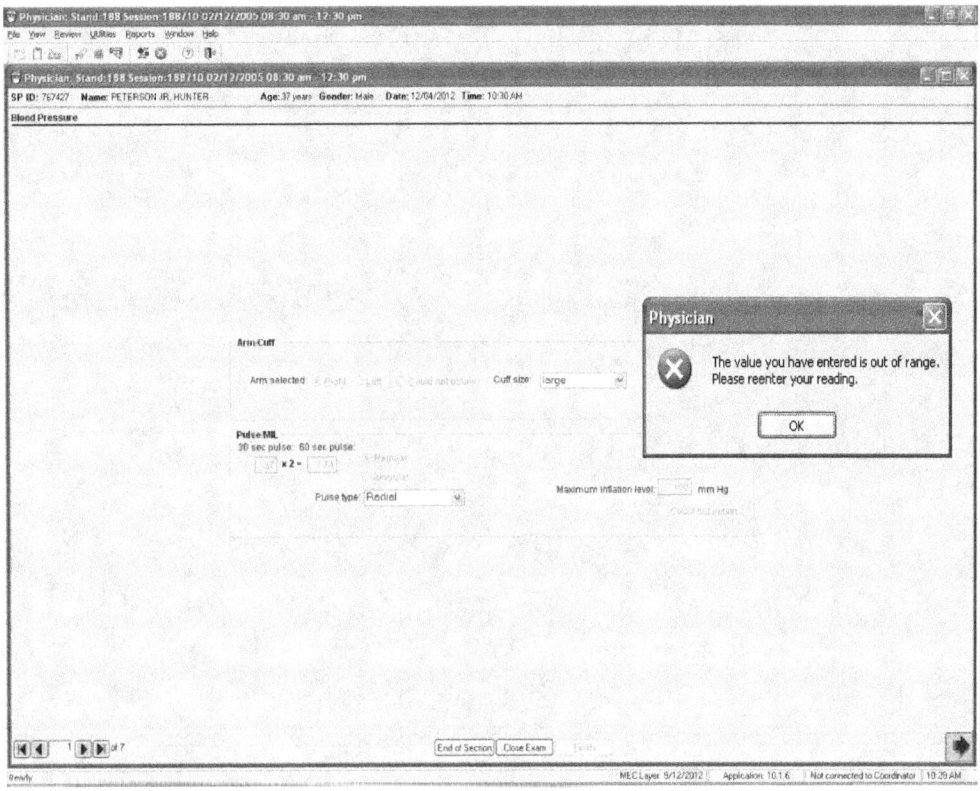

■ Alternatively, if the MIL is too low, the application will display the same hard edit alert.

■ If the Next button is entered before the MIL is entered, the system will display a message: "Please enter MIL or check "Could not Obtain." If "Could not Obtain" is selected for MIL, an attempt should be made to get a blood pressure measurement (Exhibit 3-13).

Exhibit 3-13. MIL data entry required

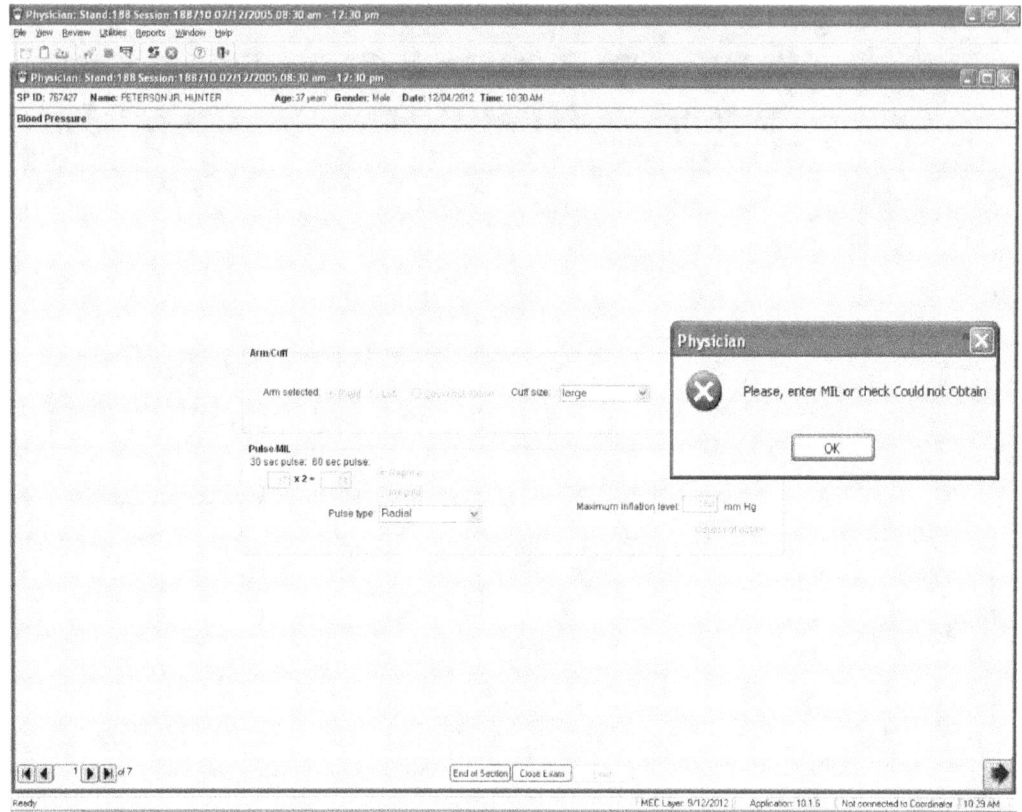

3.2 Blood Pressure Measurement Screens

■ Blood pressures are measured three times with a 30-second pause between each successive measurement.

■ If you cannot get a blood pressure measurement, check "Could not Obtain" for that measurement.

■ If the blood pressure is difficult to hear, enhancement methods may, and should, be used. See Section 3.1.4 for a description of these methods. If the enhancements are used, click on the "Enhancement" button for that measurement.

- Each BP measurement is recorded on a new screen. Advance the screen after each successive BP measurement. Do not go back to review previous BPs before taking the next measurement (Exhibit 3-14).

Exhibit 3-14. Default blood pressure data entry screen 1

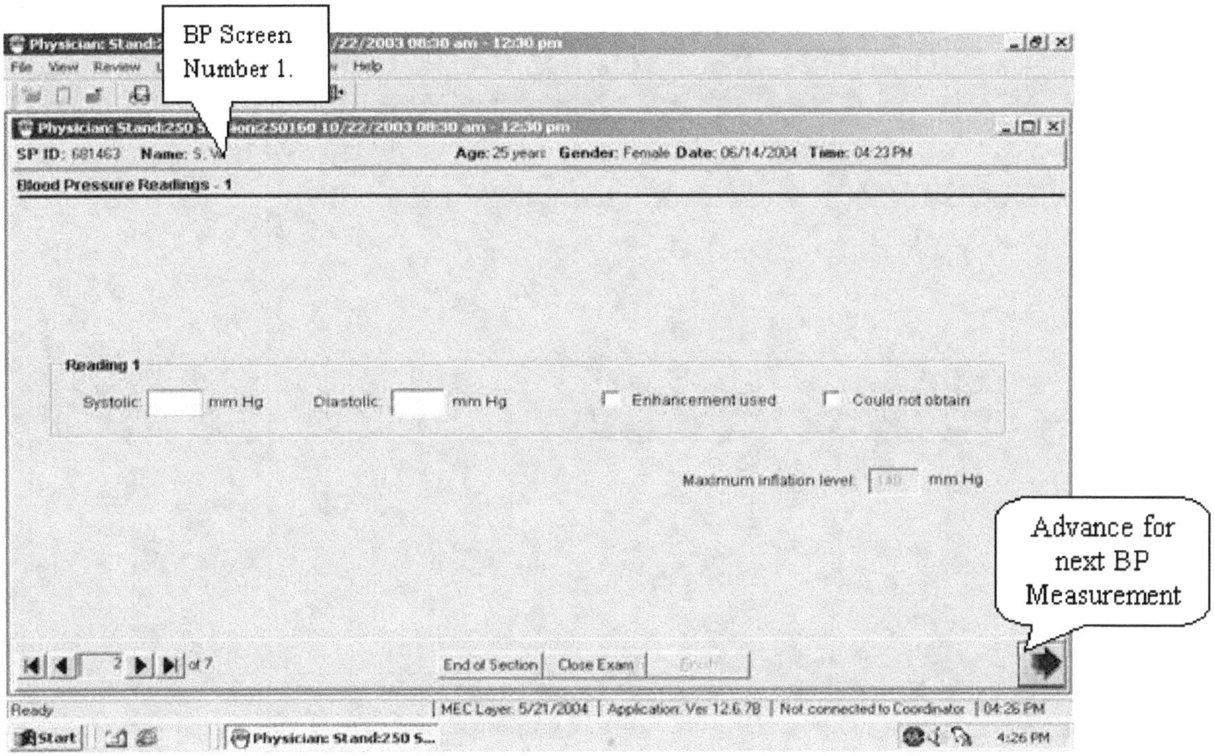

- Take the second BP using the same techniques as BP 1.

- Record the 2nd BP, and advance the screen.(Exhibit 3-15).

Exhibit 3-15. Blood pressure readings screen 2

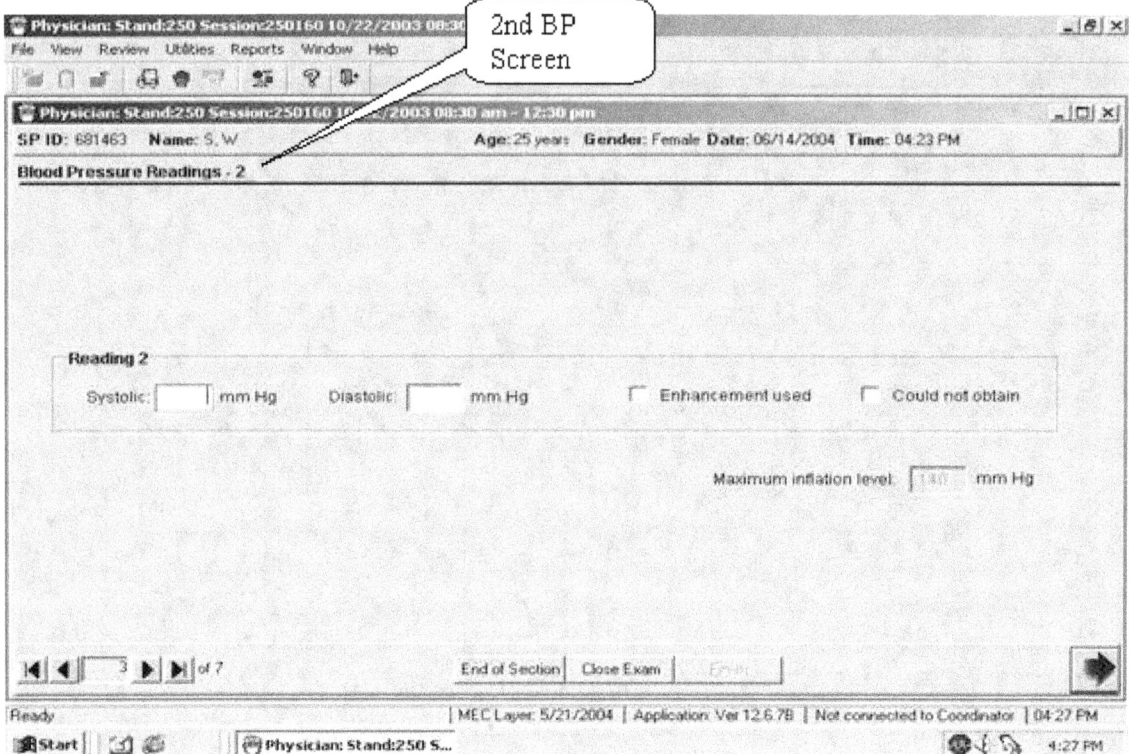

- Take the third BP using the same techniques as BPs 1 and 2.

- Record the 2nd BP, and advance the screen.(Exhibit 3-16).

Exhibit 3-16. Blood pressure readings screen 3

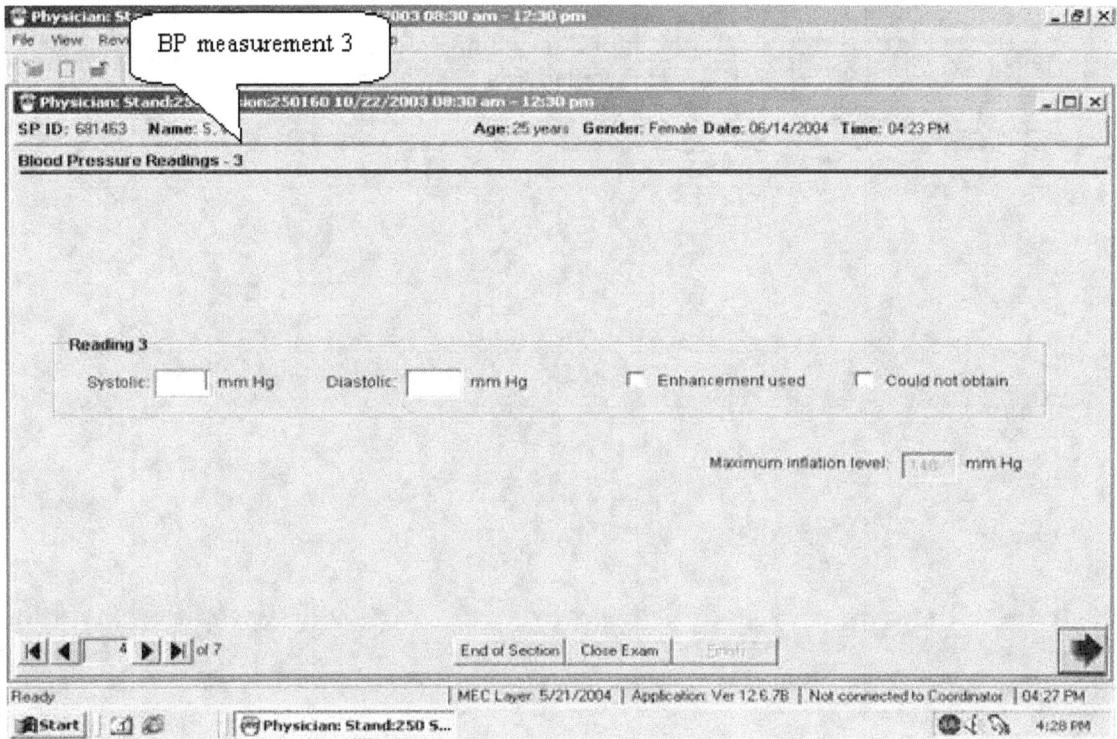

- If any of the first three measurements are checked as "Could not Obtain," the BP section of the application will open up another field to allow a fourth measurement.

- Take the fourth measurement and record the results (Exhibit 3-17).

Exhibit 3-17. Blood pressure readings screen 4

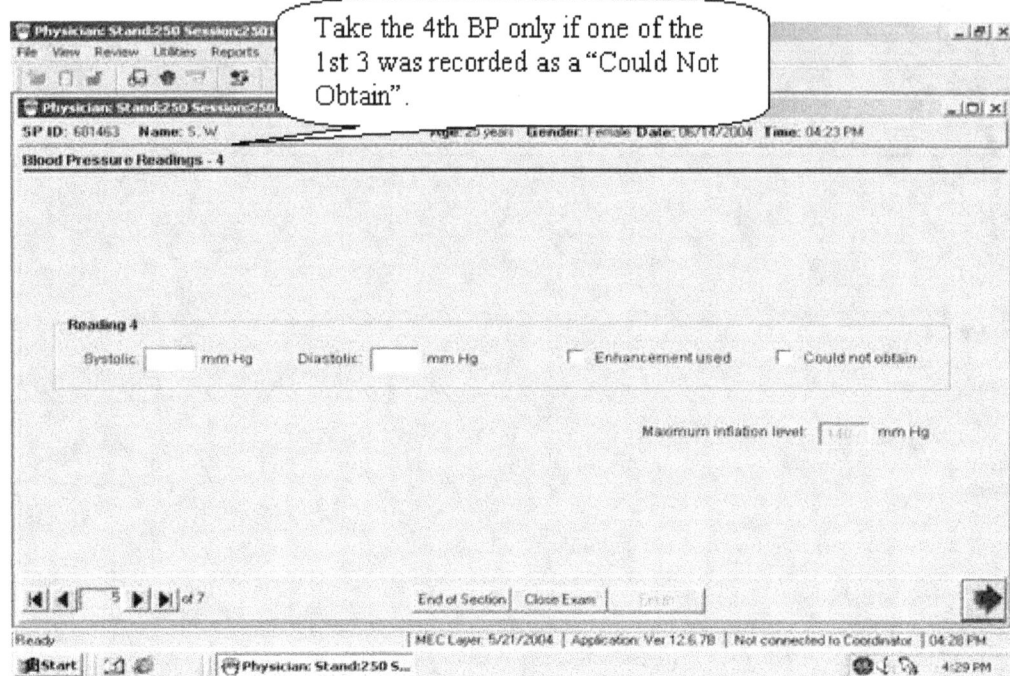

- Inflate the cuff up to five times for blood pressure measurements, including all MIL measurements.

- The increment of the mercury manometer markings are in 2-millimeter intervals. All end digit BP measurements should be recorded as even numbered digits. If an odd number is entered as the end digit for either the systolic or diastolic measurement, a message is displayed: **"Number must be even!"**

- Click OK to this message. Reenter the correct measurement and continue with data entry or measurement.

- If the systolic BP entered is greater than the MIL, a message is displayed: "SBP should be less than MIL. Please redo your MIL."

- Redo the MIL and record. The cuff can be inflated up to five times.

- There must be a MIL recorded for every SP.

- Ideally, every SP has three blood pressure measurements recorded.

- When three systolic blood pressure readings are recorded, the systolic average is calculated by the system as the average of the **last two systolic measurements.(Exhibit 3-18).**

- When only one systolic blood pressure reading can be obtained, the one systolic reading is calculated by the system as the average.

- When only two systolic blood pressure readings can be obtained, the first systolic reading is discarded and the second systolic blood pressure measurement is calculated by the system as the systolic average.

- If all diastolic readings are zero, the average diastolic BP is calculated by the system as zero (0).

- If there is one diastolic reading of zero and one or more readings with a diastolic above zero (0), the system uses only the nonzero diastolic readings to calculate the average diastolic BP.

- If two of three diastolic readings are zero (0), the system uses the one nonzero diastolic reading to calculate the average diastolic BP.

- When the average BP appears, tell the SP his or her BP.

Exhibit 3-18. Averaging systolic blood pressure

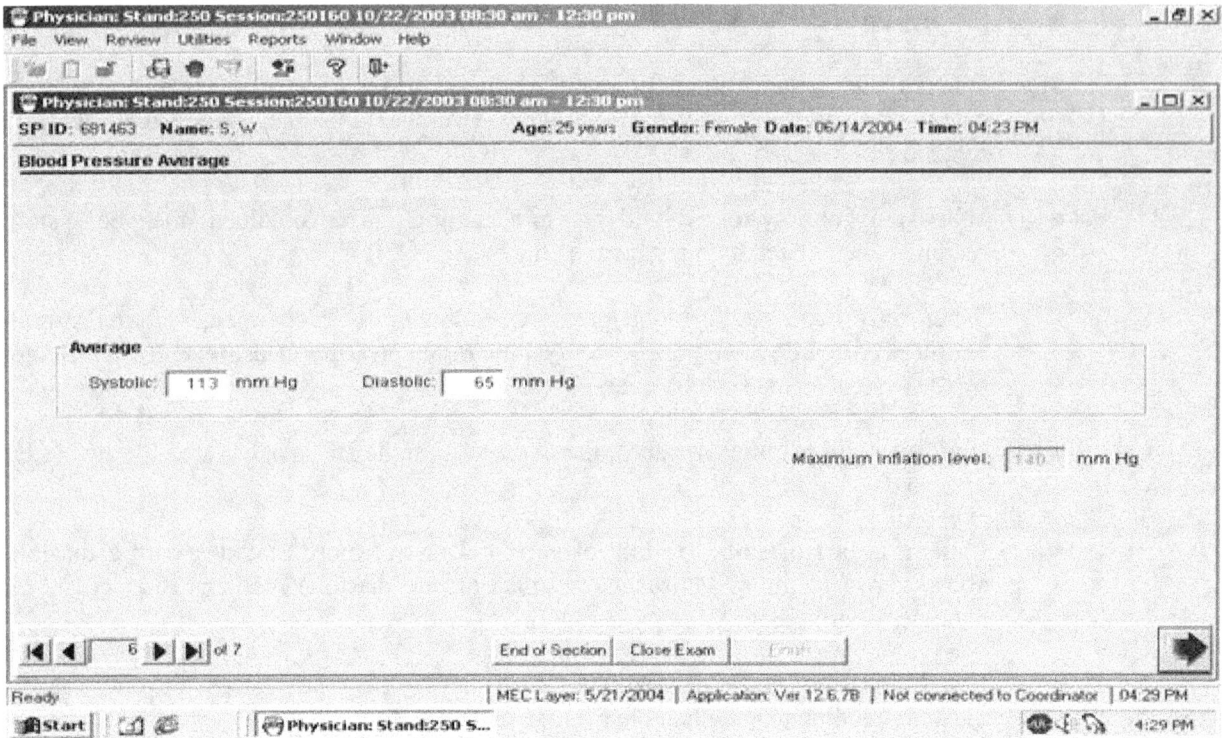

- If the systolic and diastolic BP are less than 20 mm Hg or more than 100 mm Hg, the application edits asks for verification of accuracy (Exhibit 3-19).

- If the measurements are correct, click "Yes."

- If the measures are incorrect, click "No," and reenter the measurements.

Exhibit 3-19. Edit allowable systolic and diastolic blood pressure

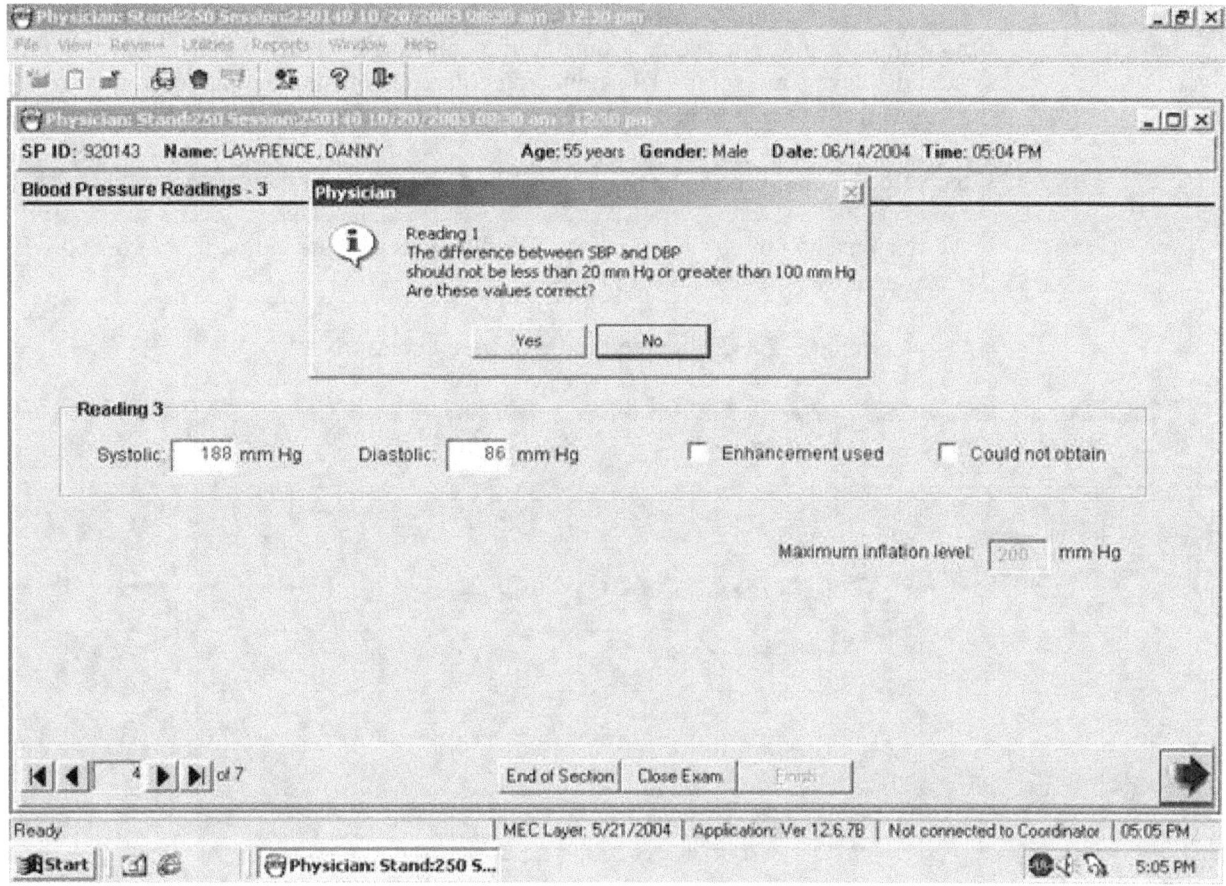

3.2.1   Blood Pressure Edit Limits

- If a systolic or diastolic value is outside the edit range for that SP, (age specific) the system displays a message: "The value you entered is outside the range for this age. Is this value correct?" (Exhibit 3-20).

- If the value entered is correct, click "Yes," and proceed with the data entry.

- If the response is not correct, click on "No" and reenter the value, then proceed with the examination.

Exhibit 3-20. Edit range limits for blood pressure

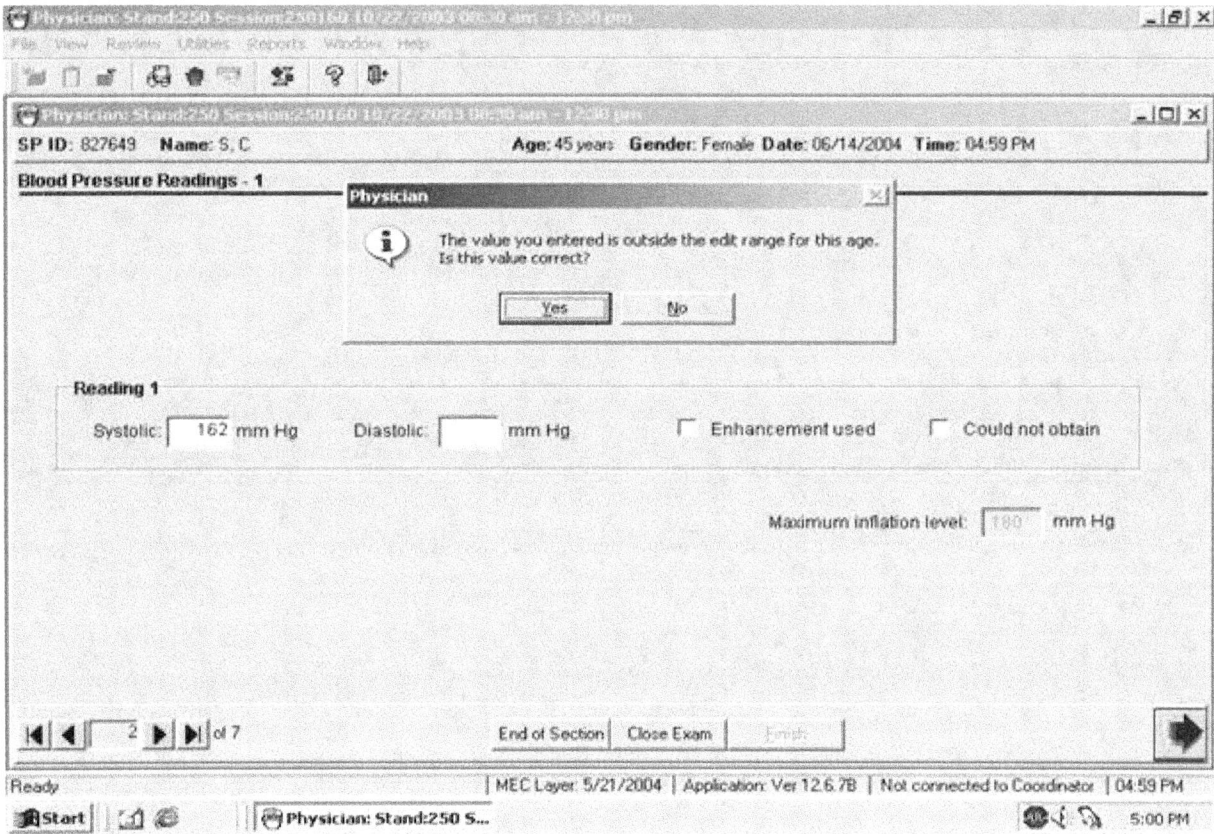

3.2.2   **Blood Pressure Component Status and Comments**

- If all the measurements were entered, the system sets the default last screen for the component status to "Complete."

- If one or more of the measurements were not recorded, the system sets the component status to "Partial."

Exhibit 3-21. Comments in blood pressure component

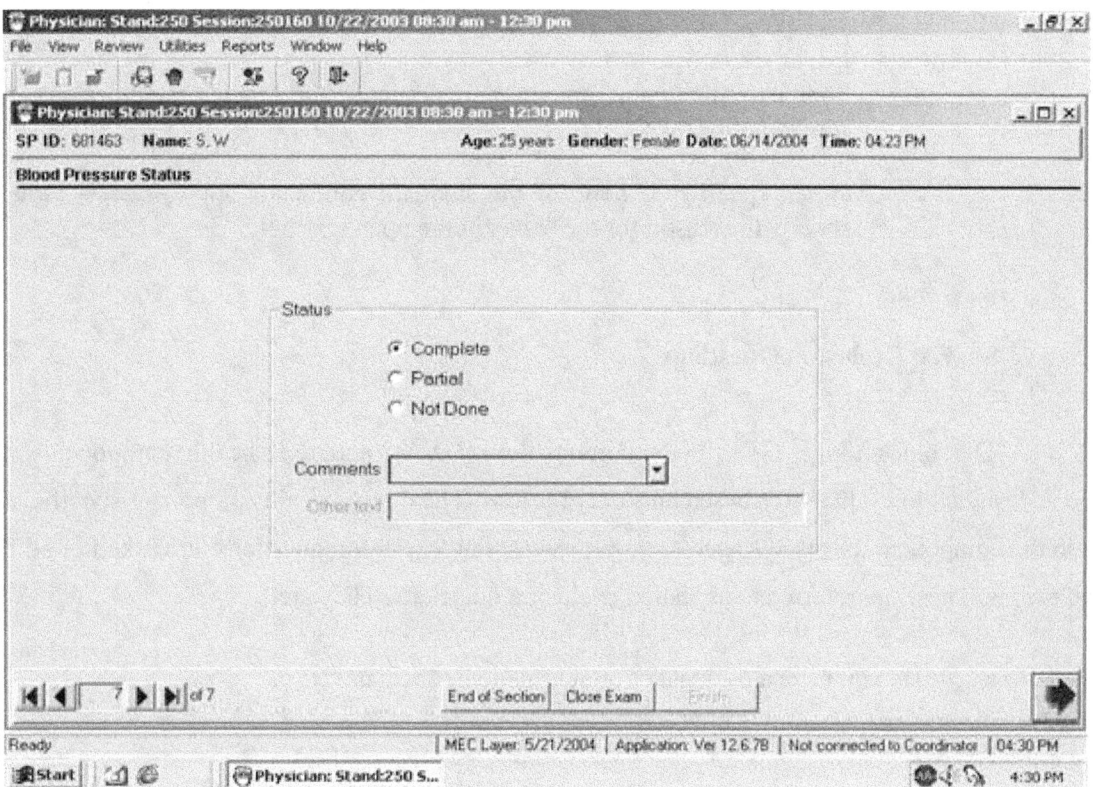

- If the Component Status is partial, select the appropriate comment from the drop-down menu.

- The comments in the menu are:

  - Safety exclusion: SP is excluded because of a situation that may cause him or her harm or discomfort such as applying or inflating a cuff on an arm with visible edema, lesions, or other conditions.

  - SP refusal: SP refuses all or part of the examination.

  - No time: SP cannot complete the examination due to time restrictions.

- Physical limitation: SP has a physical limitation that prevents examination completion.

- Communication problem: Physician cannot communicate instructions for the examination adequately.

- Equipment failure: There is a malfunction of the equipment.

- SP ill/emergency: SP became ill during the examination.

- Interrupted: Session was interrupted because of natural phenomena or other event.

- Poor cuff fit: If cuff does not fit properly, the blood pressure measurements should not be taken.

- Other, specific: If none of the standard comments apply, select "Other" and specify the reason for the status in the open text field.

3.3   Shared Exclusion Questions

The phlebotomy, GTT, body composition (DXA), and oral health components include questions designed to exclude SPs based on safety reasons. The questions are component-specific and are asked in the component for all SPs aged 16+, but two safety exclusion questions are asked of all SPs for several exams. These are referred to as shared exclusion questions. They are:

- Do you have a pacemaker or automatic defibrillator?

- Are you currently pregnant?

Safety exclusion questions that were not answered during the household interview are asked during the MEC examination at the first opportunity when the SP begins the exam. In the case of children, parents or guardians answer the exclusion questions (proxy exam) as soon as they arrive on the MEC, except for the pregnancy question. The proxy exam is conducted either by the MEC manager or the MEC interviewers. Each question is asked only once, even when the question is relevant for more than one component—this eliminates wasting time during exams to repeat questions that the SP has already answered. Note that answers to the safety exclusion questions provided during previous components will appear on the screen for the next examiner to see, but the field for data entry is disabled. Once answered, they cannot be changed.

The pregnancy question is administered to all female SPs aged 12 through 59 years. The question is also addressed to SPs aged 8 through 11 years if they reported during the household interview that menarche had begun. The physician is the only MEC examiner who asks this question.

The physician will see the two shared exclusion questions on the Shared Exclusion Screen.

■ If the SP is female, there are shared exclusion questions on self-reported pregnancy.(Exhibit 3-22).

Exhibit 3-22. Shared Exclusion Questions for females aged 12 to 59

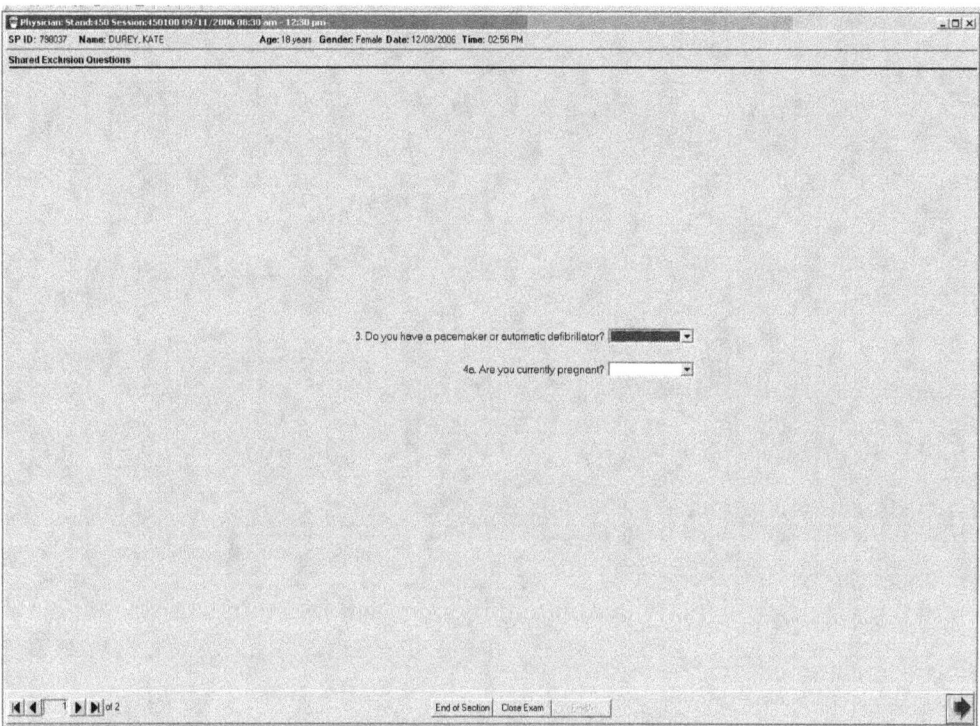

■ If the shared exclusion questions are answered in the household examination, the questions will appear answered and disabled. These responses cannot be changed in the MEC.

- This screen represents the condition in which a parent would have answered the pacemaker or automatic defibrillator question during the proxy exam, but the pregnancy question is asked by the physician during the physician exam (Exhibit 3-23).

Exhibit 3-23. Shared Exclusion Questions answered during a previous exam

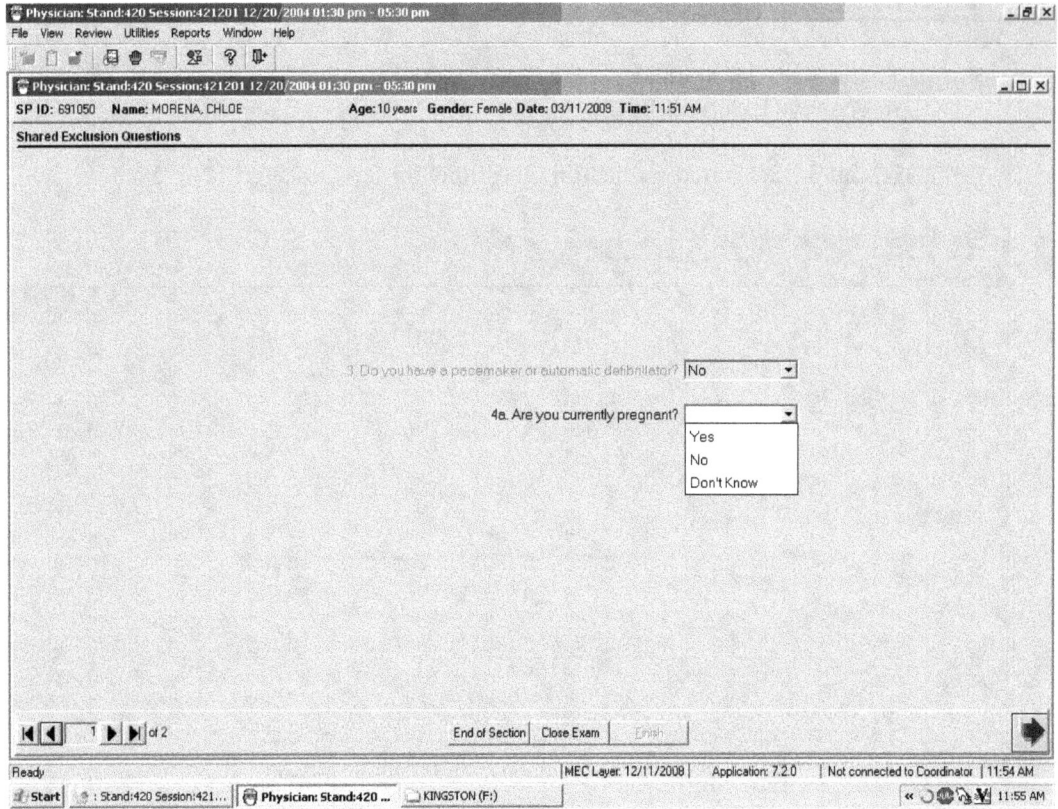

- If the pregnancy question is answered Yes, a dialogue box will appear with a message that the SP is excluded from DXA. (Exhibit 3-24).

Exhibit 3-24. Shared Exclusion Questions: Exclusion

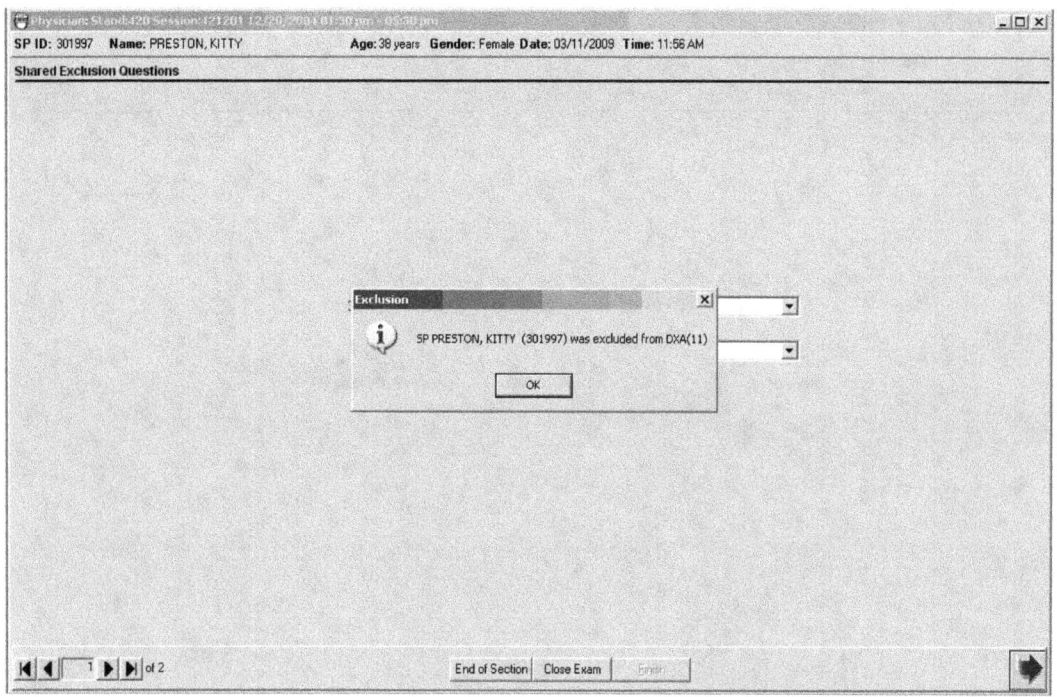

- This is the only Shared Exclusion question for SPs who are male and for females who are not of childbearing age (Exhibit 3-25).

Exhibit 3-25. Shared Exclusion Questions: Pacemaker/Automatic Defibrillator

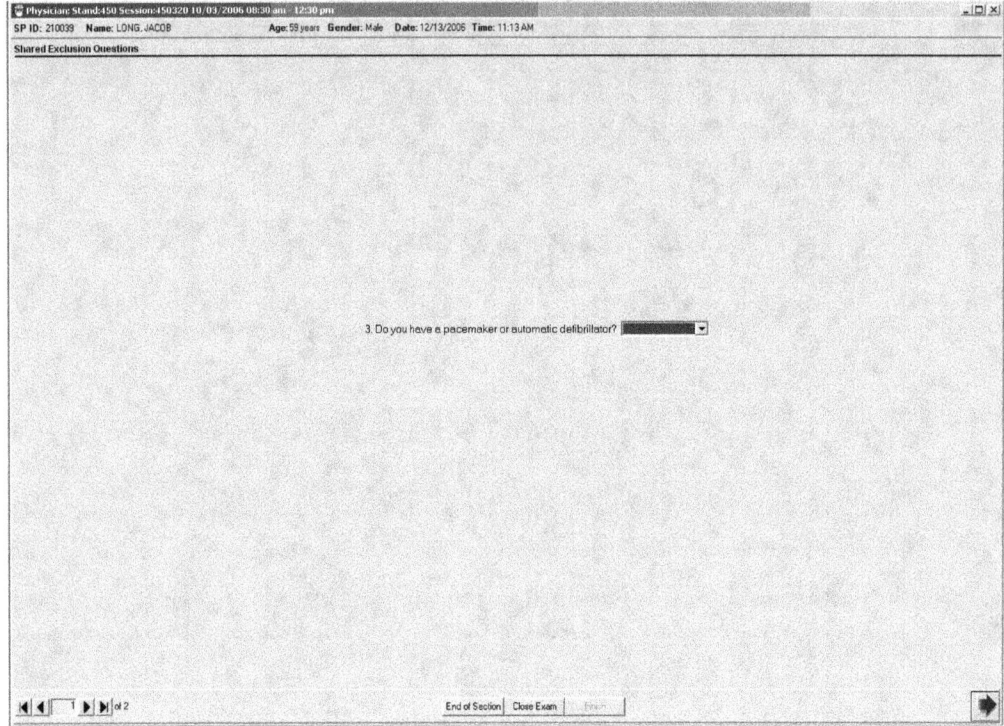

- If the Next button is pressed to go to the next screen, a message is displayed: "Please answer the question." The specific question that was not answered will also be part of this message (Exhibit 3-26).

- Click "OK" to this message and answer the question, then go to the next screen.

Exhibit 3-26. Shared Exclusion Questions: Required data entry

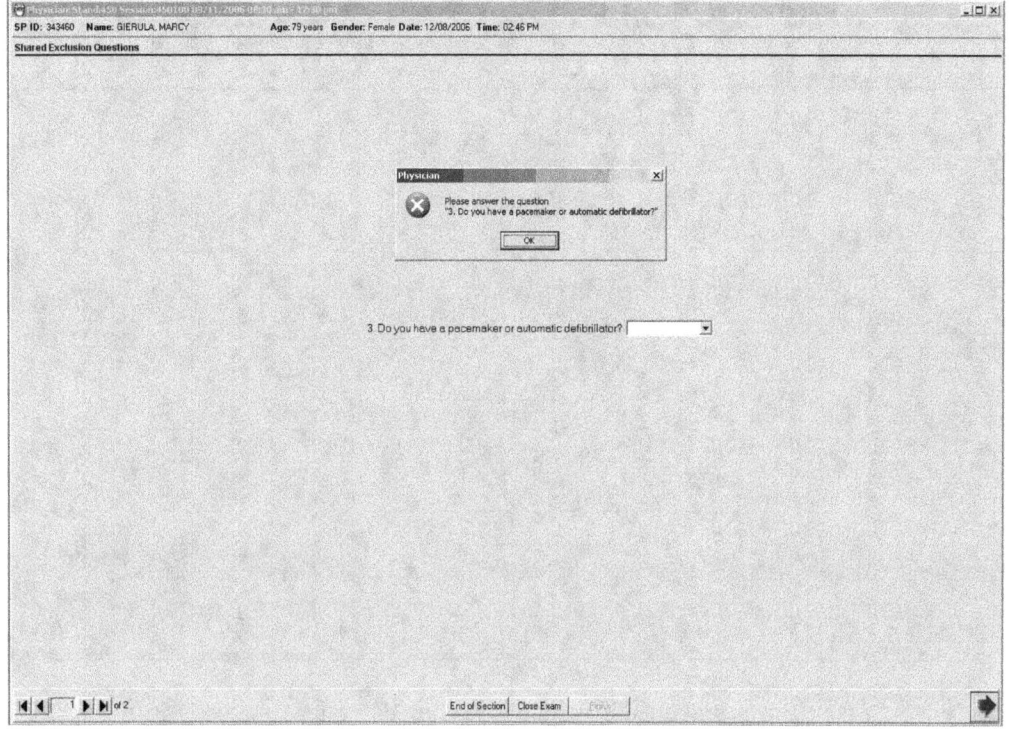

- If all the shared exclusion questions are answered, the component status for shared exclusions defaults to "Complete." (Exhibit 3-27).

- If some questions were not answered, the status defaults to partial. The examination is closed with the "Close Examination" button.

Exhibit 3-27. Component completion status for shared exclusions

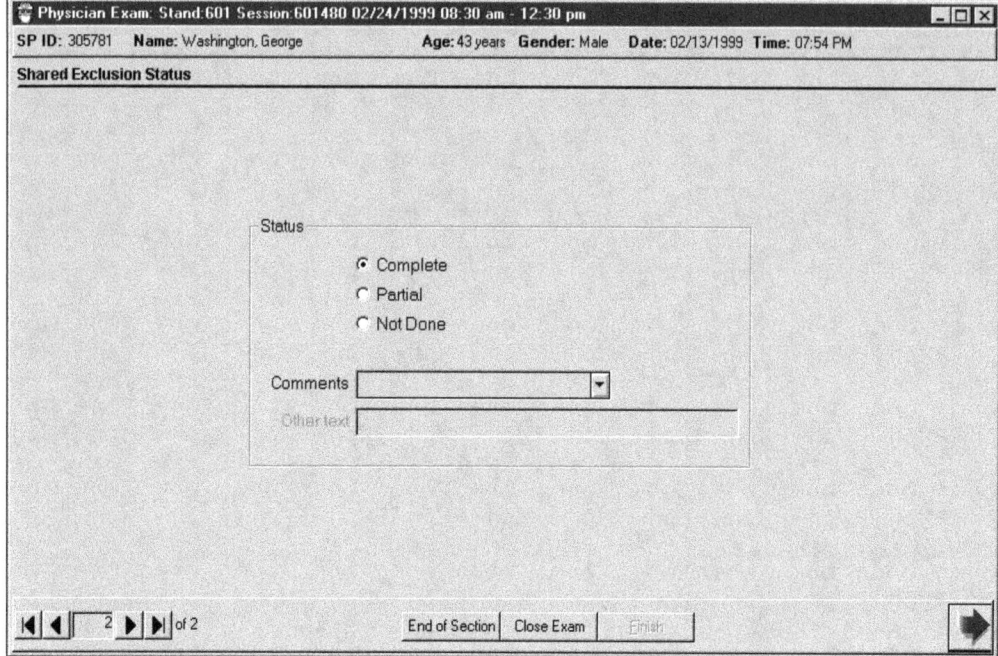

- If the SP was excluded by any of the shared exclusion questions, the system displays a series of messages to indicate the other components that are blocked for this SP.

- The SP is not excluded from DXA if the response to the question on pacemaker or defibrillator is "Yes."

- The SP is excluded from DXA if the weight is greater than 450 pounds or the height is greater than 6'5" , so the pacemaker/defibrillator question might be disabled if the SP is sent to body measures first.

3.4 Sexually Transmitted Diseases (STD) and Human Immunodeficiency Virus (HIV) Testing

During the physician's examination, age-eligible participants are informed about the STD and HIV tests conducted during the MEC examination. The physician's role is to discuss these tests with SPs, educate participants about the STD and HIV testing, and explain the mechanism for getting their personal test results. The confidential nature of the test result reports is explained. The specific tests are determined by age categories:

Test	Age	Source
Trichomonas	14 – 59	Urine
Chlamydia	14 – 39	Urine
HPV	14 – 59	Self-administered swab
Genital Herpes	14 – 49	Blood
HIV	18 – 59	Blood

The SPs consent to these tests during the household interview but may change their mind prior to the examination. Some SPs agree during the home interview but decide not to be tested when they arrive at the MEC. Other SPs do not agree to be tested during the home interview but change their mind and want to be tested when they arrive for the examination. Whatever the outcome, the examiner is responsive to the decision of the SP, and the SP must give his or her informed consent for these tests.

3.4.1 Guidelines Affecting STD and HIV Test Result Reporting

Two guidelines affect the confidential reporting of STD, HIV, and HPV test results to participants in NHANES. First, NHANES is not subject to state laws that require reporting STD results to state health departments. Second, adolescents in the United States can consent to the confidential diagnosis and treatment of STDs. Medical care for these conditions can be provided to adolescents without parental consent or knowledge. Therefore, there is no legal obligation to disclose findings to anyone other than the participant (CDC, *1993 Sexually Transmitted Diseases Treatment Guideline*, MMWR 42 RR-14).

STD and HIV test results are confidential and are **not disclosed to anyone,** including the participant's doctor, insurer, family, or friends except at the SP's specific request and **only** after the SP properly provides the password selected during the examination. Everyone working with the NHANES signs a legal document making them subject to the Privacy Act, the Public Health Service, and other laws.

Because of the medical, social, and emotional consequences of positive STD and HIV tests, disclosure of results is always handled in a sensitive, respectful, and confidential manner. SPs can obtain their results only when they call the toll-free telephone number provided to them during the examination. STD and HIV tests results are the only NHANES SP health examination results that are provided verbally. All other findings from the health examination are reported to persons in a written report that is mailed to them. The methods for reporting results of these tests differ slightly for adolescents and adults, as well as for non-English speaking Asians whose interviews were conducted in Chinese (Simplified & Traditional), Korean, and Vietnamese. These methods are described in the following sections.

3.4.1.1   Instructing SPs How to Obtain Confidential Test Results

SPs are instructed to call the National Center for Health Statistics personnel for their password- protected confidential reports. Test results are not provided unless the caller correctly states the password. Under no circumstances are STD test results put in writing with a respondent's name, address, or any other personal identifiers. Test results are communicated only by telephone specifically and solely to the SP.

To assure that these results are provided only to the SP for whom they are specified, SPs are asked to provide their own password. Participants are more likely to remember a password that they have selected. Physicians record the password in the physician application and inform participants that they must call a toll-free number to get their individual results. SPs use their personally-selected password to confirm their identity when they call for their results. The physician encourages SPs to keep their password confidential and not share the information with anyone.

All SPs receive a reminder notice (Exhibit 3-28) that includes the toll-free number, the date 30 days after the exam date when the results will be available, and their password. Adult participants (aged 18 years and older) receive their reminder notice from the coordinator as they leave the MEC. The reminder notice is in an envelope that is handed directly to the SP along with the Preliminary Report of Findings.

Minors (SPs 14-17 years) receive the same reminder notice but, instead of receiving it at checkout from the coordinator, the physician personally places the form in a sealed envelope marked with a number that was previously placed on the SP's examination gown. (When SPs change into an examination gown at the beginning of the session, they are given a numbered basket in which to store clothing. The assistant coordinator marks the number of the basket on the gown for subsequent identification). The physician gives the envelope to the assistant coordinator who places it in the SP's numbered basket. The physician reminds the SP to retrieve the envelope from the basket when changing clothes to leave the MEC.

Exhibit 3-28. Reminder form to get STD, HIV, and HPV results

National Health and Nutrition Examination Survey
STD AND HIV CALLBACK REMINDER

How to get results for sexually transmitted diseases and HIV

Call toll free: **1-888-301-2360**

When: **anytime after 8/3/1999**

Hours: **Monday – Friday, 8:30 am – 6:00 pm Eastern Time**

When calling for results, you will need to provide the following information:

Sample Number: 955543

Password: Picture

We will only give results to the person tested.

Participants who do **not** call for their report are sent a letter reminding them to call the toll-free number to receive their special test results. If they do not call the survey, staff from NCHS will contact them by phone and tell them their results, whether positive or negative. If a health problem is identified, the participant is informed and referred for treatment in his or her local area.

Non-English speaking Asian languages

If the language at interview was Chinese (Cantonese or Mandarin), Korean or Vietnamese, instruct the SP to provide a password consisting of digits only (numerals). The instruction letter for STD test results differs from the English/Spanish instructions as follows:

National Health and Nutrition Examination Survey

How to get your sexually transmitted disease (STD) test results:

You will be called by a NHANES Health Educator after *<insert date: 28 days after the exam>*. There will be an interpreter on the line who speaks your language.

When we call you, please provide the password below. We will only give results to the person tested.

Password: 78392

Additional Guidance for Limited English Proficient (LEP) Participants: Telephonic Interpretation

The National Health and Nutrition Examination Survey contracts with a telephonic interpreter service provider to enhance confidential communication with Limited English Proficient (LEP) participants. The service should be limited to confidential discussions that the physician wishes to conduct with the participant when the participant and/or the physician is uncomfortable with the local person serving as interpreter. For example, a male interpreter might be considered culturally inappropriate for confidential discussions regarding STDs, instructions for the vaginal swab, or pregnancy with a female. Some locally hired casual interpreters may not be able to interpret medical terminology. Or the discussion may be of such a sensitive nature, such as depression screening, that using a friend or family member to conduct such a mental health assessment would be inappropriate.

The service is available "24/7/365" and guarantees connection to an interpreter in 30 seconds. It is essential to provide no personally identifiable information *except for the SP's first name.*

Following is the protocol for using the service. Laminated instruction cards are provided for a quick reference.

Telephonic Interpretation on the Mobile Examination Center

1. When you determine that Pacific Interpreter services are needed, explain to the SP (and the local interpreter) that you are going to call a professional interpreter service to help you communicate the health-related topic(s) you wish to discuss with her/him.

2. Check the cordless handset to make sure it is functional and that you have a dial tone.

3. Using your wall telephone, call the toll-free number:

4. Provide the CDC – FIELD Access Code:

5. Ask for the language you need and explain that the participant is in the room with you. The operator will connect you to an interpreter.

6. Script for the introductory discussion (before giving SP the handset) with the interpreter only:

   I am Dr. _____. I work with a national health survey. I have a participant here in the room with me, and I would like to discuss _____(your topic)_____ with her/him.

   Now I am going to give a second headset to the participant, __(participant's first name)_____.

7. Continue with your discussion with the participant using the NHANES interpreter protocol but, most importantly, speak in short sentences to the interpreter and address the participant directly.

Table 3-3 summarizes the STD/HIV testing protocol.

Table 3-3. Summary table of STD/HIV testing protocol

Age	Protocol
SPs ages 14 - 17	• English and Spanish speakers select their password in any combination of letters/digits. • Non-English Asian language speakers select their password in *numerals only*. • Physician enters the password into the application • Physician prints the letter, places it in an envelope while SP is still in room. The physician does not write any personally identifiable information on the letter or envelope except for the belongings basket number. • The letter is placed with SP's basket of belongings and is retrieved directly by the SP when she or he changes back into street clothing. The letter is not intended for any other individual.
Ages 18 - 59	• English and Spanish speakers select their password in any combination of letters/digits. • Non-English Asian language speakers select their password in *numerals only*. • Physician enters the password into the application. • The reminder letter is printed with the Checkout Package at the coordinator station when the SP leaves the examination center.
14–59 English and Spanish speakers	• English and Spanish speakers are instructed on the reminder letter to call for results in 30 days. • If the SP has not called for the results, a text message will be sent on days 38, 48, and 58. • The test message will read: "Reminder: Please call 888-301-2360 to get your password- protected test results from the health survey."
14–59 Non-English speaking Asians	• Instruct SP that a representative from NCHS will contact him or her by telephone when results are ready after 30 days; • SP must provide his or her selected password when the representative calls.

3.4.2　　　Gaining Cooperation for the Female HPV Swab

Women ages 14-59 are asked to provide a vaginal swab for human papillomavirus (HPV) testing. The swab is self-collected by the women in the privacy of the bathroom after receiving instructions from the physician. The next sections describe the vaginal swab protocol.

The physician will explain the HPV assessment after discussing the tests for sexually transmitted diseases and HIV and then obtaining participant's password. The following is the suggested physician script.

Instructions

"We ask all girls and women your age to participate in a test for human papillomavirus. You may not have heard about these conditions. Human papillomavirus is sexually transmitted and many women who are infected do not have any symptoms.

We test for HPV using vaginal fluid. I will explain how to collect a vaginal specimen yourself. Here is a kit that contains one vaginal swab, smaller than a tampon. You will do this in the bathroom where you will have complete privacy. I recommend that you wash your hands before starting and after completing the collection. Also, because you will be inserting a swab into your vagina, you may want to undress partially before starting. Once you are ready to begin, first twist the top off the clear soft plastic tube. Do not discard the top. Place the top on a clean surface. Remove the swab from the plastic tube. Hold the stick at the end and do not touch the foam part of the swab. Hold the lips of the vagina open with one hand. Insert the swab fully into the vagina (like a tampon) with your other hand. Turn the foam swab against the walls of your vagina as you count to 10. Carefully remove the swab without touching the skin or hair outside of the vagina. Place the swab in the soft plastic tube and replace the cover on the tube. When you are done, you can give the tube to the staff person who will be waiting outside the bathroom. There are written instructions in English and Spanish inside the package if you need a reference."

Instructions for women in the third trimester of pregnancy vary in that the SP is instructed to insert the swab halfway into the vaginal area by holding the swab about halfway from the end of the swab.

"Do you have any questions about this test?"

"How do you feel about taking part in this test?"

(If participant indicates she is uncomfortable, you can probe "you seem unsure about doing this; what are you thinking about?" Remember the participant has the right to refuse this test. If the participant refuses this test, explain, "This will not affect your participation in the rest of the study.") If the participant agrees to the test, explain:

"Like the blood and urine tests that are being done, these results are very private, and we will give these results only to you. We will not put the results in the report that is mailed to your home. We will give you a toll-free number to call in 4 weeks, and results will be reported only after you provide the password which you gave me a few minutes ago *<password provided during STD/HIV pretest counseling>.*"

3.4.3 Gaining Cooperation for the Male HPV Swab

Boys and men within ages 14-59 are asked to provide a penile swab for human papillomavirus (HPV) testing. The swab is self-collected by the men in the privacy of the bathroom after receiving instructions from the physician. The next sections describe the penile swab protocol.

The physician will explain the HPV assessment after discussing the tests for sexually transmitted diseases and HIV and then obtaining participant's password. The following is the suggested physician script.

Instructions

We ask men (boys) your age to collect a specimen to test for human papillomavirus, also called HPV. HPV is sexually transmitted and many men (boys) are infected but do not have any symptoms. This test isn't routinely done in the doctor's office so we won't be giving you the results of this test.

We're going to go over how you will collect the specimen **yourself**. First you do not have to put the swab inside your penis. You just need to rub the soft tip of a swab on the outside of your penis.

Let's look at these diagrams and go through the steps.

- You will do this in the bathroom **alone** where you will have complete privacy

- Because you will be rubbing the swab on the penis, you will need to undress partially and wash your hands before starting.

- Once you are ready to begin, first twist the top off the plastic tube. Do not throw away the top. Place the top on a clean surface facing up (SHOW DIAGRAM).

- Remove the swab from its package. Hold the swab about 2 inches from the soft tip, but do not touch the soft tip of the swab. Hold your penis and **firmly rub** the soft tip of the swab on your penis several times. You should rub vigorously* on all sides so that the entire surface of the penis is touched by the swab. This includes the top surface, both sides, and under the penis. This should take about 10 seconds (count slowly 1, 2, 3….10)

- If you are uncircumcised (point to uncircumcised illustration) pull the foreskin back and firmly rub the surface under the foreskin as well.

- Then place the soft tip of the swab in the plastic tube; bend the swab shaft at a 90 ^{0} angle against the side of the tube and break the stick.

- Put the top back on the tube tightly (SHOW DIAGRAM).

- When you are done, place the tube in the rack.

There are written instructions inside the package if you need help.

Followup questions may be required in order to gain the SP's cooperation in this collection:

"Do you have any questions about this test?"
"How do you feel about taking part in this test?"

(If participant indicates he is uncomfortable, you can probe "you seem unsure about doing this; what are you thinking about?" Remember that the participant has the right to refuse this test. If the participant refuses this test, explain, "This will not affect your participation in the rest of the study.") If the participant agrees to the test, explain:

"Like the blood and urine tests that are being done, these results are very private, and we will give these results only to you. We will not put the results in the report that is mailed to your home. We will give you a toll-free number to call in 4 weeks, and results will be reported only after you provide the password which you gave me a few minutes ago *<password provided during STD/HIV pretest counseling>*.

3.4.4   Testing for Trichomonas

With the SP's consent, testing for the presence of the STD trichomonas will be done for SPs aged 14-59 from their urine sample. While the other STDs may be somewhat familiar to the SP, trichomonas will likely be less well known, so the physician needs to be prepared to provide some background and explanation of the disease and its treatment. Results of the testing will be reported to the SP in the same manner as the other STDs.

3.4.4.1   Talking Points

Here are some talking points the physician can use to explain the cause, transmission, and effect of the trichomonas infection.

- Trichomoniasis (or "trich") is a very common sexually transmitted disease that is caused by infection with the protozoan parasite Trichomonas vaginalis. Although symptoms of the disease vary, most women and men who have the parasite cannot tell they are infected.

- Trichomoniasis is considered the most common curable STD. In the United States, an estimated 3.7 million people have the infection, but only about 30 percent develop any symptoms. Infection is more common in women than in men, and older women are more likely than younger women to have been infected.

- The parasite is passed from an infected person to an uninfected person during sex. In women, the lower genital tract (vulva, vagina, or urethra) is most commonly infected. In men, the most commonly infected body part is the inside of the penis (urethra). During sex, the parasite is usually transmitted from a penis to a vagina, or from a vagina to a penis, but it can also be passed from a vagina to another vagina. It is not common for the parasite to infect other body parts, such as the hands, mouth, or anus. It is unclear why some people with the infection get symptoms while others do not, but it probably depends on factors like the person's age and overall health. Infected people without symptoms can still pass the infection on to others.

- About 70 percent of infected people do not have any signs or symptoms. Symptoms of trichomoniasis can range from mild irritation to severe inflammation. Some people develop symptoms within 5 to 28 days after being infected, but others do not develop symptoms until much later. Symptoms can come and go.

- Men with trichomoniasis may feel itching or irritation inside the penis, burning after urination or ejaculation, or some discharge from the penis.

- Women with trichomoniasis may notice itching, burning, redness or soreness of the genitals, discomfort with urination, or a thin discharge with an unusual smell that can be clear, white, yellowish, or greenish.

- Having trichomoniasis can make it feel unpleasant to have sex. Without treatment, the infection can last for months or even years.

- Trichomoniasis can increase the risk of getting or spreading other sexually transmitted infections. For example, it can cause genital inflammation that makes it easier to get infected with the HIV virus, or to pass the HIV virus on to a sex partner.

- It is not possible to diagnose trichomoniasis based on symptoms alone. For both men and women, your primary care doctor or another trusted health care provider must do a check and a laboratory test to diagnose trichomoniasis.

- Trichomoniasis can be cured with a single dose of prescription antibiotic medication (either metronidazole or tinidazole), pills which can be taken by mouth. It is okay for pregnant women to take this medication. However, some people who drink alcohol within 24 hours after taking this kind of antibiotic can have uncomfortable side effects.

- About one in five people who have been treated get infected again within 3 months after treatment. To avoid getting reinfected, make sure that all of your sex partners get treated too, and wait to have sex again until all of your symptoms go away (about a week). Get checked again if your symptoms come back.

- Using latex condoms correctly every time you have sex will help reduce the risk of getting or spreading trichomoniasis. However, condoms don't cover everything, and it is possible to get or spread this infection even when using a condom.

- The only sure way to prevent sexually transmitted infections is to avoid having sex entirely. Another approach is to talk about these kinds of infections before you have sex with a new partner so that you can make informed choices about the level of risk you are comfortable taking with your sex life.

3.4.5   Discussing STD and HIV Testing and Instructing the SP How to Obtain Results

The exhibits in this section show how the physician discusses STD and HIV testing with different age groups and how he or she instructs the SP to obtain results.

If the SP is 14-17 years of age, the physician discusses the method for the SP to receive STD results.

Exhibit 3-29. STD Tests for SPs 14-17 years old

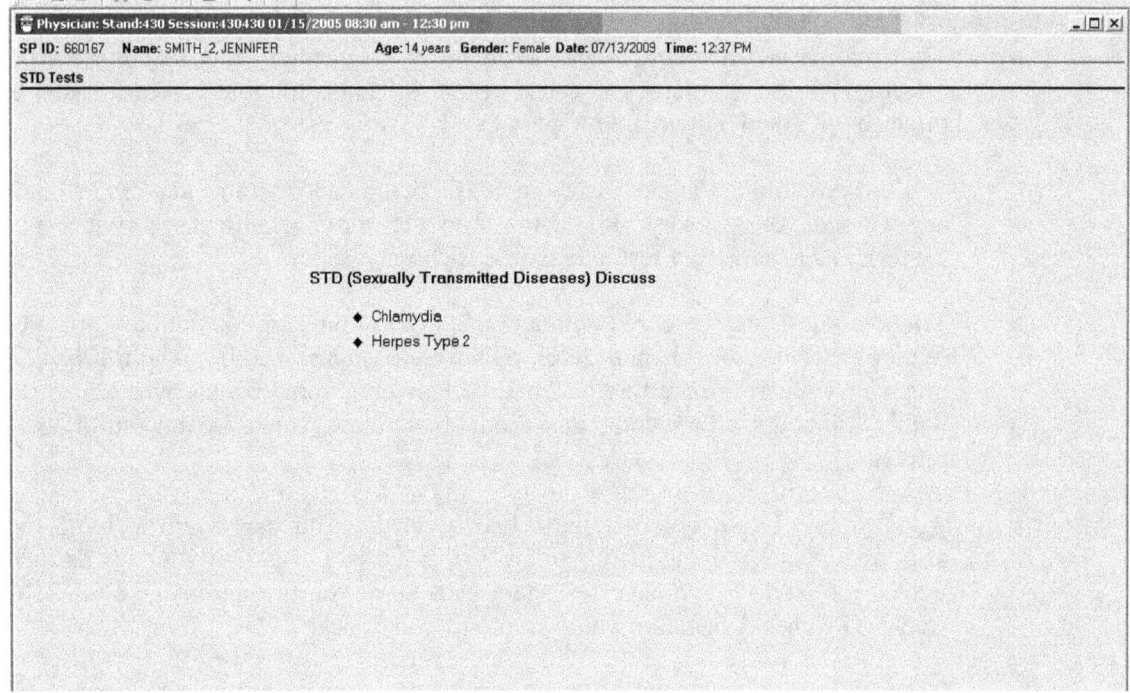

Exhibit 3-30. STD password field for 14 year old

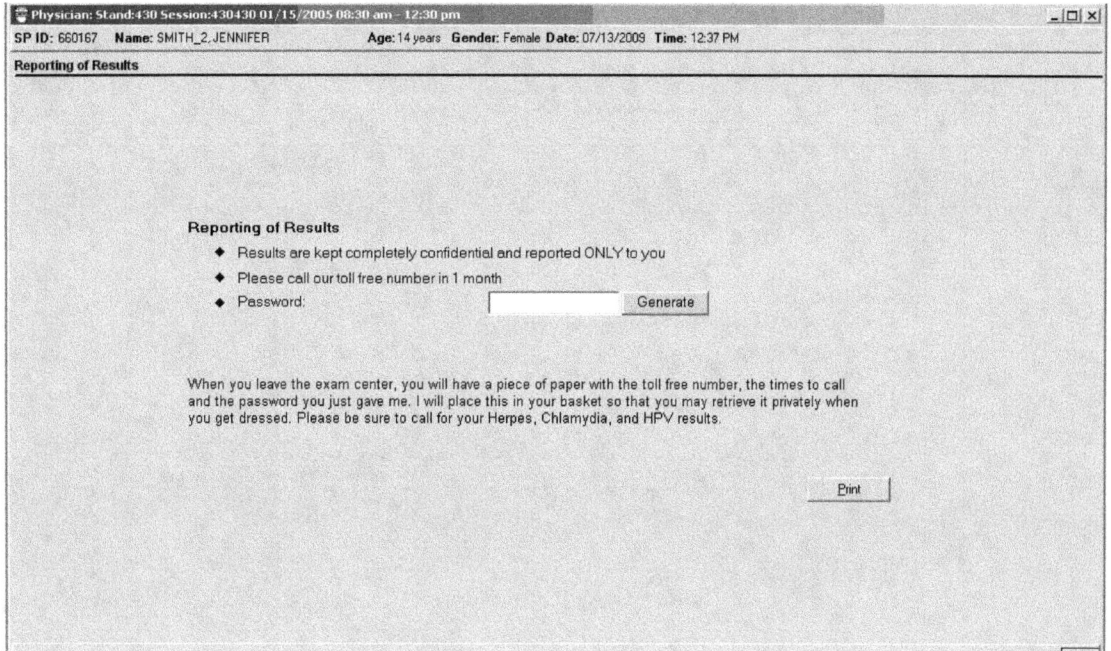

- The physician asks the SP to give a password to use when calling to get his or her test results. If the SP cannot think of a password, the physician will give the SP a password by clicking on "Generate" (Exhibit 3-31). The system will generate a password and display it in the password field. Physicians are discouraged from application-generated passwords, as the SP is more likely to forget that password and may misplace or discard the instruction form. Be patient with the SP while he or she thinks of a password.

Exhibit 3-31. STD password automatically generated

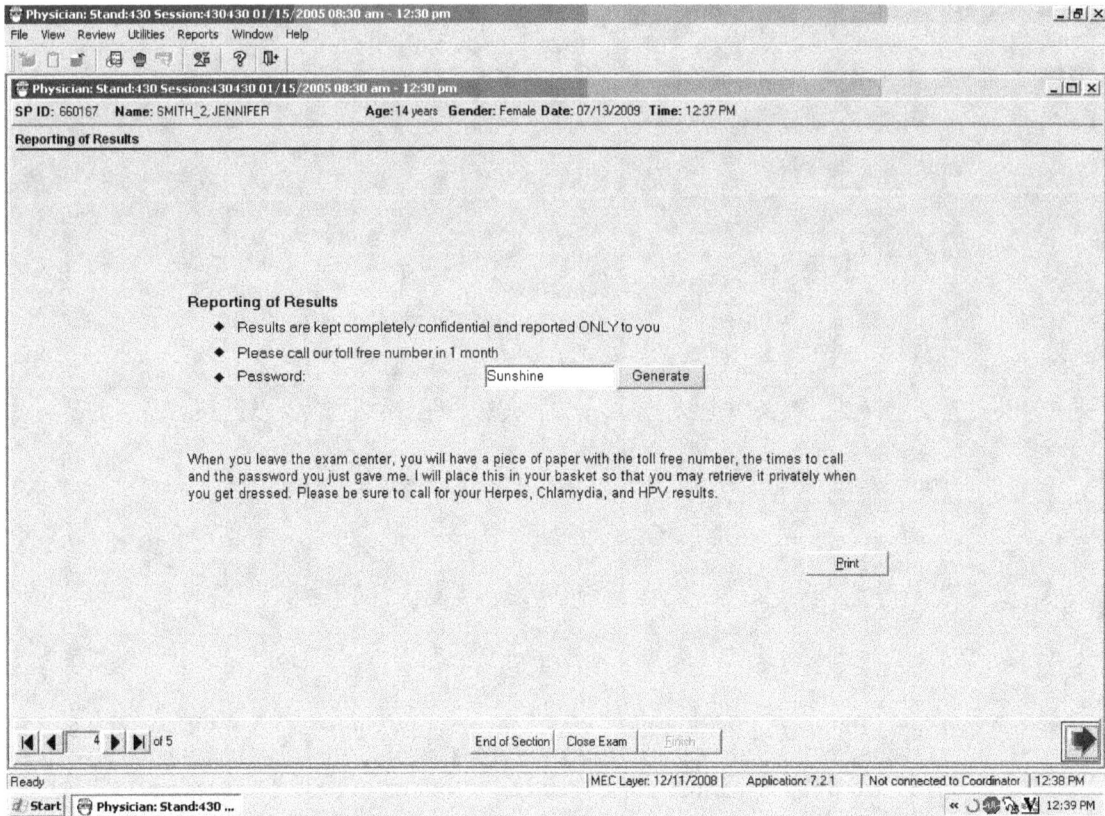

- Other SP information on minors is given to the parents at the time of checkout from the MEC. Because of the sensitive and confidential nature of STD results, the information reports for 14- to 17-year-olds are printed in the physician's room and the test results are given only to the SP.

- Click on the "Print" button to print the information form for the SP. After discussing the mechanism for obtaining test results, put the STD and HIV information form in a sealed envelope.

- On the envelope, write the number on the SP's examination gown (the number corresponding to the number on the basket containing the SP's clothes). Put the envelope in your mailbox or give it directly to the assistant coordinator who will put the envelope in the basket corresponding to the number on the envelope.

- If the SP is 18-39 years of age, the physician discusses the method for the SP to receive results for STD and HIV (Exhibit 3-32).

Exhibit 3-32. STD and HIV for SPs 18-39 years old

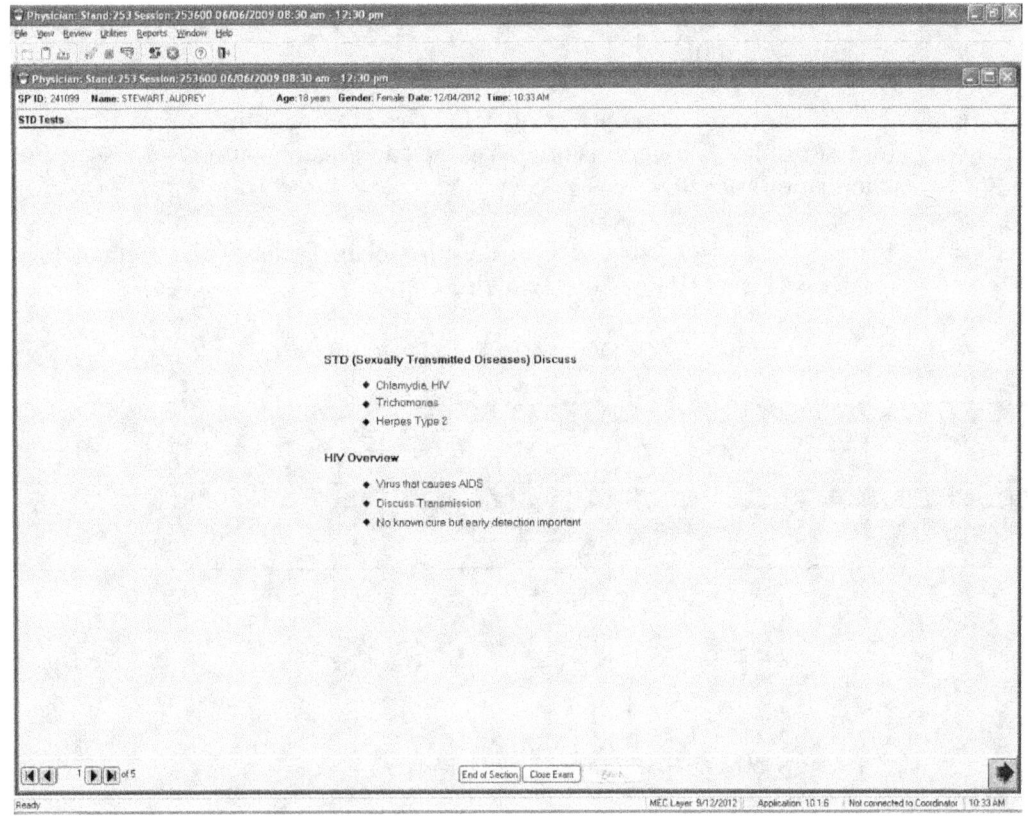

- The physician asks the SP to give a password to use when calling to get the test results. If the SP cannot think of a password, the physician will give the SP a password by clicking on "Generate." The system generates a password and displays it in the password field.

- The SP is given a printout during MEC checkout with the information needed to call for test results. The form is printed at the coordinator station and placed with the SP's information packet.

- If the SP is 40-49 years of age, the physician discusses the method for the SP to receive STD and HIV results. Exhibit 3-33).

Exhibit 3-33. STD and HIV for SPs 40-49 years old

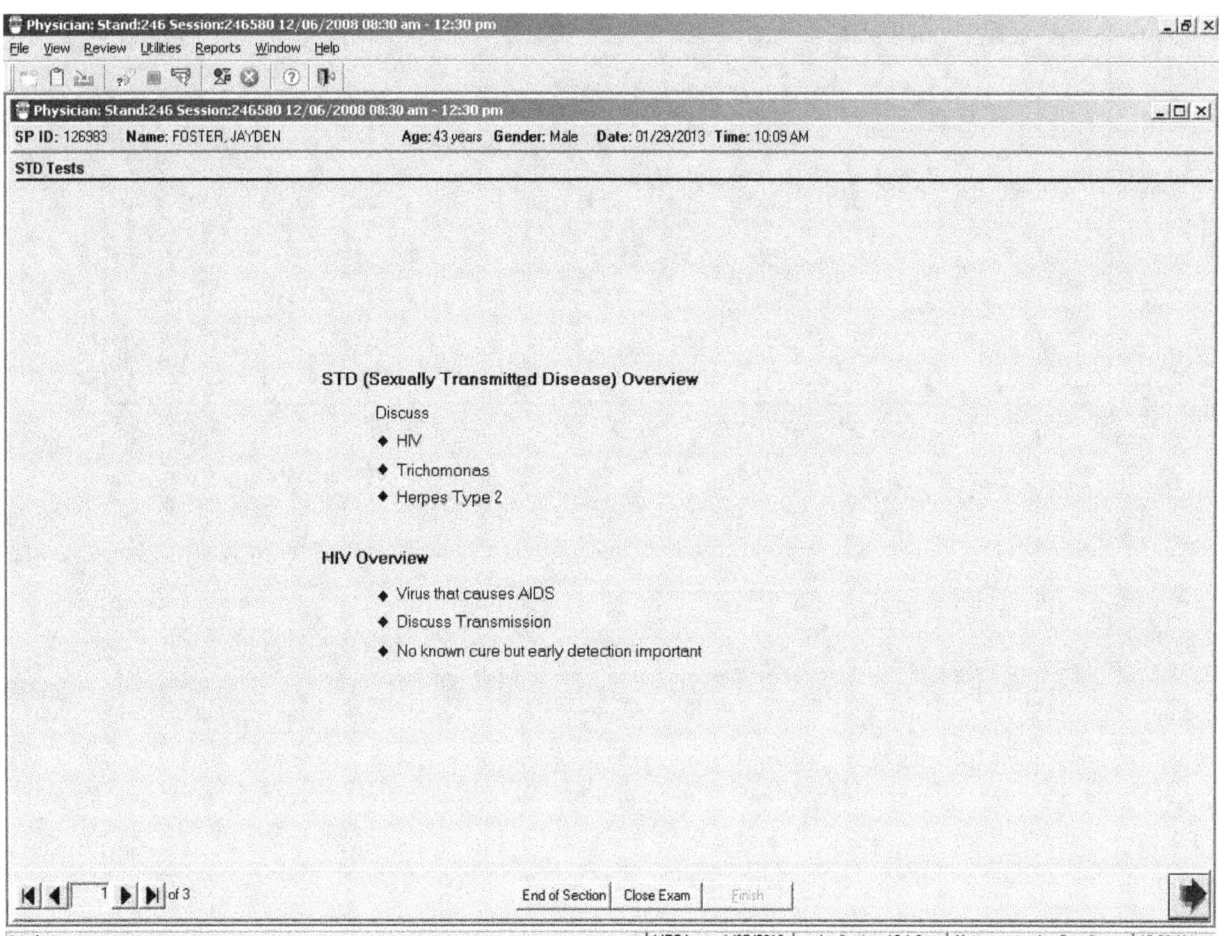

- The physician asks the SP to give a password to use when calling to get test results.

- If the SP cannot think of a password, the physician will give the SP a password by clicking on "Generate."

- The system generates a password and displays it in the password field.

- The SP is given a printout at the time of MEC checkout with the information needed to call for test results. This form is printed at the coordinator station and placed with the SP's information packet.

- If the SP is 50–59 years of age, the physician discusses the method for the SP to receive HIV results (Exhibit 3-34).

Exhibit 3-34. STD and HIV for SPs 50 - 59 years old

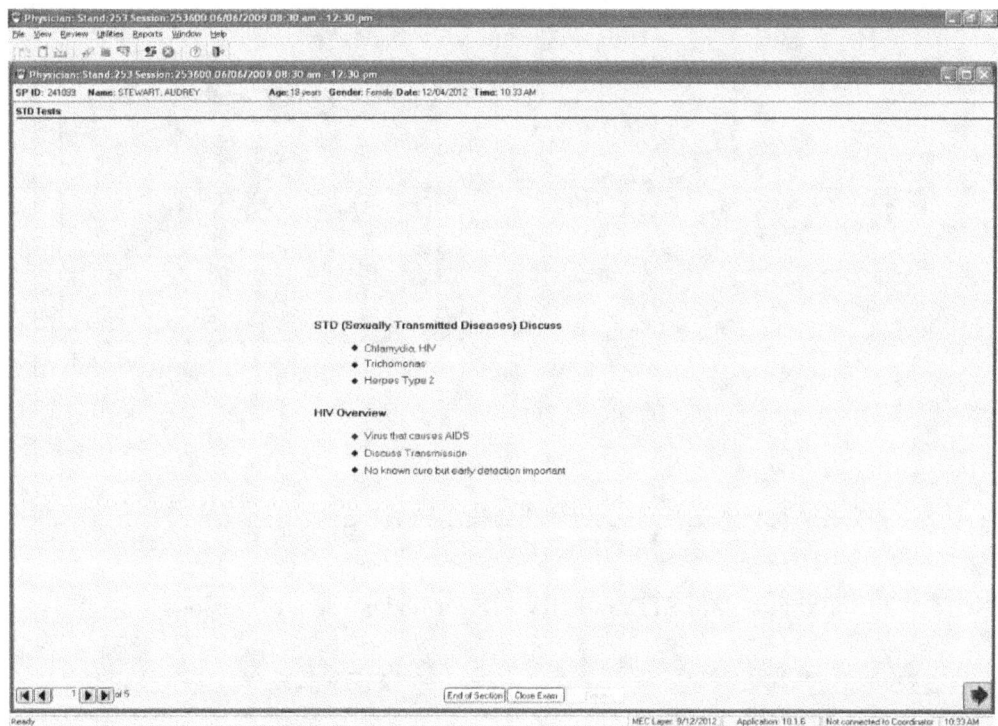

- The physician asks the SP to give a password to use when calling to get test results. If the SP cannot think of a password, the physician will give the SP a password by clicking on "Generate." The system generates a password and displays it in the password field.

- The SP is given a printout at the time of MEC checkout with the information needed to call for test results. This form is printed at the coordinator station and placed with the SP's information packet.

3.4.6   Informed Consent Designation in ISIS

SPs may refuse the STD and/or the HIV tests. They may do this during the household interview or in the phlebotomy room. The SP can also be excluded for STD and or HIV during the physician's examination or at any time during the visit to the MEC. If the SP determines that he or she wants to refuse any or all of these tests, the physician accesses the "Utilities" menu from the toolbar and selects "IC Exclusions" (Informed Consent exclusions) (Exhibits 3-35 and 3-36).

Exhibit 3-35. Utilities menu for informed consent exclusions

Exhibit 3-36. STD and HIV – Informed consent exclusions

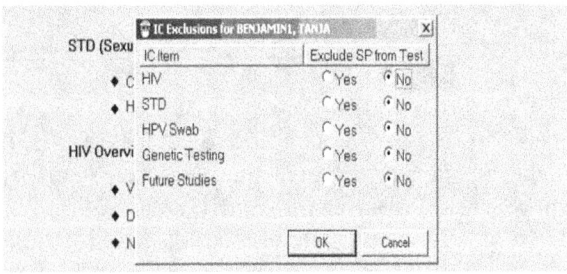
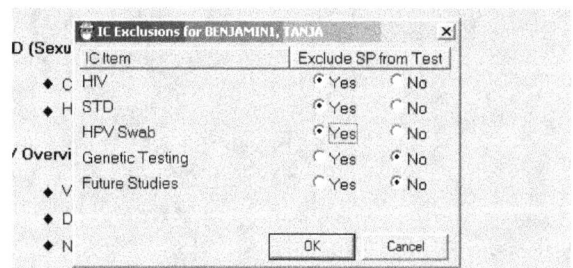

- If the SP had previously agreed to these tests and later decided to refuse these tests after discussion with the physician, the specimens can be still be excluded. Select "Yes" to exclude the SP from HIV, STD, or HPV swab tests. This sends a message to the phlebotomy and laboratory examination component to exclude the SP from these tests.

- The SP could refuse these tests initially and later change his or her mind after talking with the physician or phlebotomist. In this situation, the informed consent exclusion should be unchecked. This will remove the exclusion for these tests in the laboratory.

- If the SP refused to have STD and HIV testing either during the consent process or in the phlebotomy room, the screen in the physician's examination appears with a message over each section that was refused: "Participant has refused STD and HIV testing." (Exhibit 3-37).

Exhibit 3-37. SP refusal for STD and HIV testing

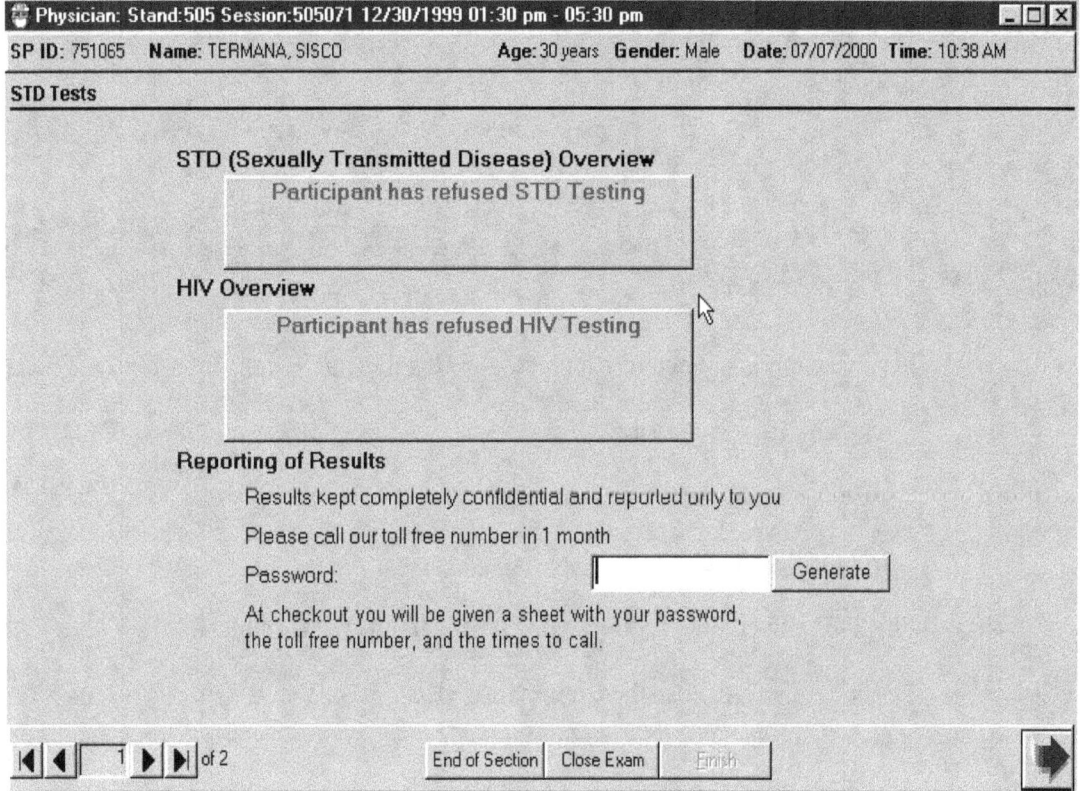

- If the SP refuses the testing, it is not necessary to discuss the mechanism for getting results. It is not necessary to have the SP select a password. Select the "Next" button to go to the component status.

Exhibit 3-38. Password entry requirement for STD and HIV

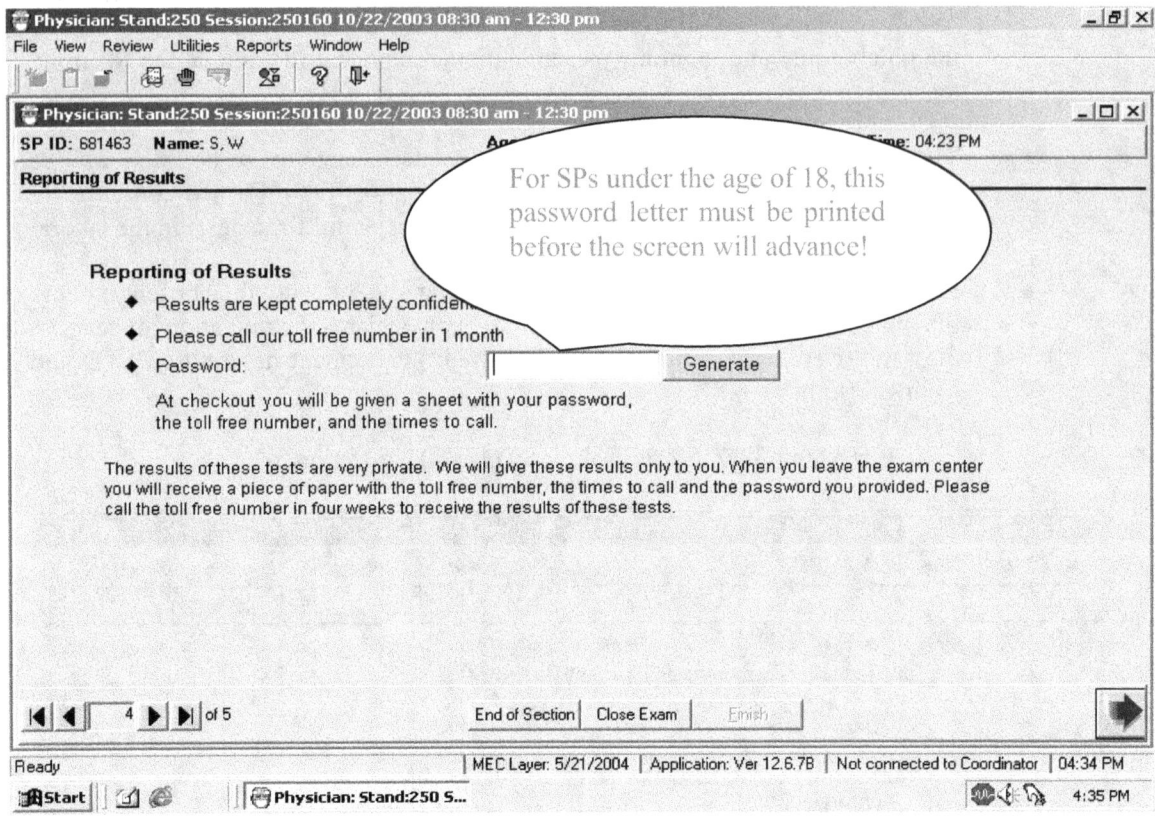

- If a password is not entered, a message is displayed: "Please enter the Password."

- Click "OK" to this message.

- Generate a password if one is needed.

- Select the "Next" button to go to the next screen.

- The STD and HIV test completion status defaults to "Complete."

- Select "Finish" to close the examination (Exhibit 3-39).

Exhibit 3-39. STD and HIV test completion status

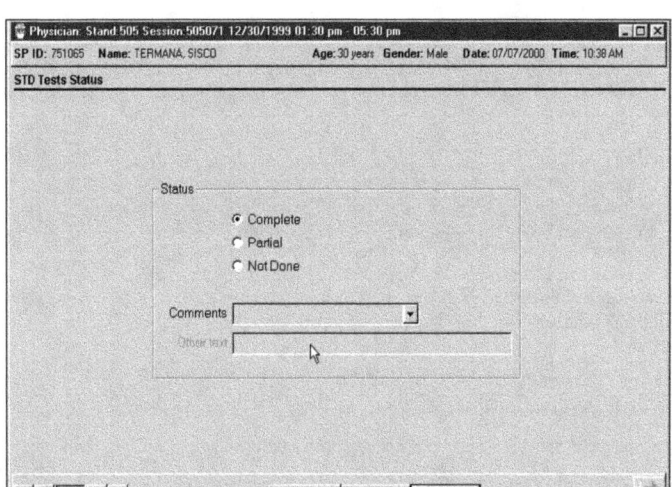

3.5 The Physicians' Role in the Pubertal Maturation Interview Informed Consent

The physician's role in supporting the pubertal maturation component of the MEC interview is not a direct function of the physician exam protocol, but it is vital role in enhancing the response rates of this interview. The pubertal maturation informed consent exclusion is accessed through the physician application, and this section explains the physician's responsibility in supporting the consent process.

A Pubertal Maturation self-assessment is administered in the ACASI section of the MEC Interview to SPs aged 8-19. Because of the sensitive nature of the topic, it is introduced during the Automated Proxy exam to the parent/guardian of minors and explained with the aid of a flyer designed for parents. Before SPs aged 18 are assigned to the MEC Interview, a parent/guardian will be informed during the Automated Proxy Interview that his or her child will be asked questions about body development and is given the flyer to read. Below is the script used in the proxy interview to introduce the pubertal maturation section of the MEC Interview, followed by the flyer that is given to respondents (Exhibits 3-40 and 3-41).

Exhibit 3-40. Script for proxy interview

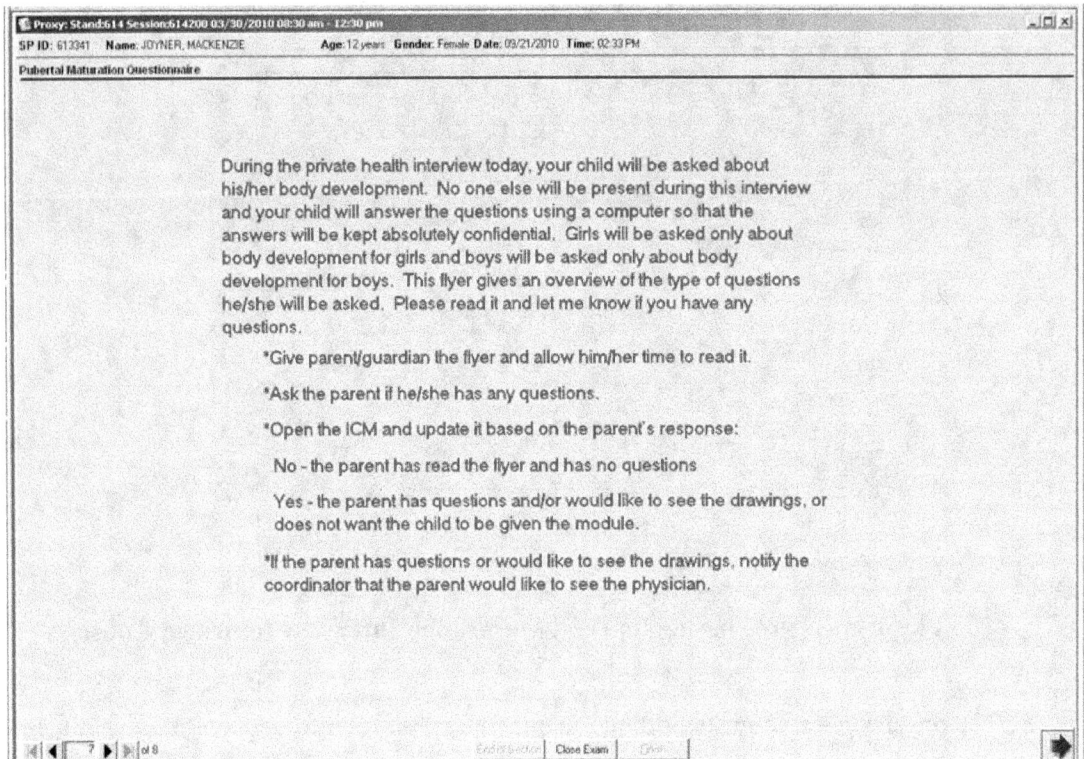

During the private health interview today, your child will be asked about his/her body development. No one else will be present during this interview and your child will answer the questions using a computer so that the answers will be kept absolutely confidential. Girls will be asked only about body development for girls and boys will be asked only about body development for boys. This flyer gives an overview of the type of questions he/she will be asked. Please read it and let me know if you have any questions.

> *Give parent/guardian the flyer and allow him/her time to read it.

> *Ask the parent if he/she has any questions.

> *Open the ICM and update it based on the parent's response:

> No - the parent has read the flyer and has no questions

> Yes - the parent has questions and/or would like to see the drawings, or does not want the child to be given the module.

> *If the parent has questions or would like to see the drawings, notify the coordinator that the parent would like to see the physician.

Exhibit 3-41. Flyer given to respondents for the pubertal maturation section

NHANES Body Development Questions

During the private health interview in the NHANES mobile examination center your child will be asked about his or her body development.

The questions we ask in NHANES about body development help us to know if a child is in the early, middle or late stage of puberty – the time when children develop into adults. We know that children grow and develop at different ages. This is normal.

During the private interview, your child will be asked about his or her body development stages using a touch screen computer. No one else will be in the room. We use drawings that show the stages of body development during puberty. We ask girls to pick drawings of the pubic hair and breast development stages that look most like their bodies. Boys will be asked to pick drawings of the pubic hair and genital development stages that look most like their bodies. Girls will see only drawings of girls' development stages and boys will see only drawings of boys' development stages. The doctor in the mobile examination center has copies of the drawings we use in NHANES if you would like to see them.

Every year more than 1,000 children and teens participate in NHANES. Your child's answers will be combined with answers from other children. These answers will be used with other NHANES information such as height and weight, body fat, bone health, and results from blood tests to provide very important information about child growth and development in the United States. This information will help doctors and other health professionals to better deal with health problems that may affect children.

Participation in the interview is voluntary and the information your child provides will be kept private and will not be given to anyone.

Thank you for participating in NHANES!

If the respondent decides that he or she does not want his or her child to receive the Pubertal Maturation questions, that section of MEC Interview is blocked. If a respondent feels that he or she would make a better decision with more information about the body development questions, and what the drawings look like, the interviewer offers the respondent an opportunity to meet with the physician. In this case, the proxy interviewer sets the IC exclusion to "Yes" and informs the coordinator or MEC manager that the respondent has been referred to the physician for a consultation on the body development interview.

When the respondent visits with the physician, he or she will be shown the age-appropriate drawings that the child will see in the ACASI screens. The respondent will then decide whether to have the child participate in the body development section. The physician is advised to use the following talking points to explain the body development questions.

What is puberty? Puberty is a time of many changes in body development, when girls start to grow into women and boys into men. During puberty, teens may notice acne, oily skin, growth of underarm hair, and body odor. They may put on weight, girls especially, and go through a growth spurt. Parents may notice a change in their child's emotions. These are all normal stages in growth and development.

When does puberty or changes in body development start? Changes in girls during puberty can begin anywhere between 8 and 14 years of age. Puberty in boys usually begins after the girls, between 10 and 15. But everyone matures at different ages – this is normal and one of the reasons NHANES is asking about body development stages, to find out how girls and boys in the U.S. are doing.

Why is NHANES asking about body development? The information we collect in NHANES on stages of body development is used with other information from NHANES to help provide a picture of the health of children and teens in the U.S. For example, the stage of body development is more important than actual age in determining the growth of healthy bones. The body development stage is used to look at the level of iron in the blood, an important indicator of health. Doctors and other health professionals will be able to use the information from the body development questions and other NHANES tests to plan programs to better deal with health problems facing children and teens. Body development stage is an important piece of the puzzle that health care professionals use to understand the growth and development of children and teens in the U.S.

What does NHANES do with the answers to these questions? The answers to the body development questions are combined with answers from thousands of other children and teens for use in research on the health of children and teens and the development of programs and policies. Each person's answers are kept private so that no one else will know what those answers are.

Why are drawings used? Studies have shown that, when drawings are used together with descriptions, children and teens can more accurately pick their stages of body development than if only the descriptions were used. NHANES worked with medical illustrators at the National Institutes of Health to create drawings that are accurate but appropriate for viewing by children and teens. Girls will see only drawings of girls' development stages and boys will see only drawings of boys' development stages.

Will I find out if the body development stage picked is the right one? You will not receive the results from the body development component because the results will not be as accurate as those provided by your family doctor or pediatrician. You should talk with your family doctor or pediatrician if you are concerned about body development or puberty. Physical examinations of children and teens usually include a check on pubertal status.

Why can't I go with my child to help answer the body development questions? The questions are asked privately so that children and teens can answer honestly. Teens in particular may be embarrassed and answer differently if someone else is in the room.

Why can't I have a copy of the drawings? Due to the sensitive nature of the drawings, NHANES would like them kept private and viewed only by participants and/or their parents.

3.5.1 Procedure for Changing the PM IC Exclusion

If the respondent gives verbal consent after your consultation with them, the physician must go into the PM IC Exclusion module in the Utility drop-down menu in the physician application (Exhibit 3-42) and click on PM IC Exclusion.

Exhibit 3-42. The Utilities drop-down menu displaying the PM IC Exclusion

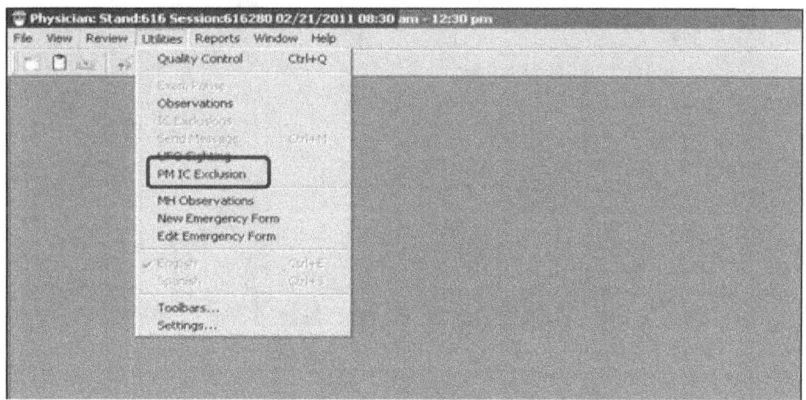

SPs who are eligible for the pubertal maturation section are displayed as in Exhibit 3-43. In this screen, only one SP is displayed. Click on the SP's name, and the IC module appears as in Exhibit 3-44. Change the "Yes" to "No," click "OK," and the module will appear in the MEC Interview for that SP.

Exhibit 3-43. List Age-Eligible SPs for Pubertal Maturation in Current Session

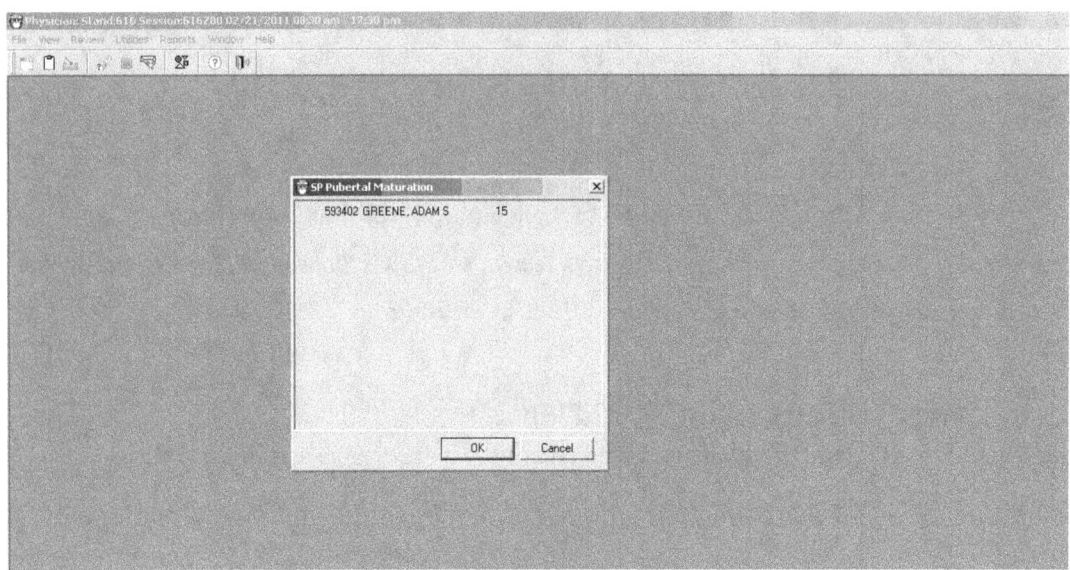

Exhibit 3-44. Pubertal Maturation Module

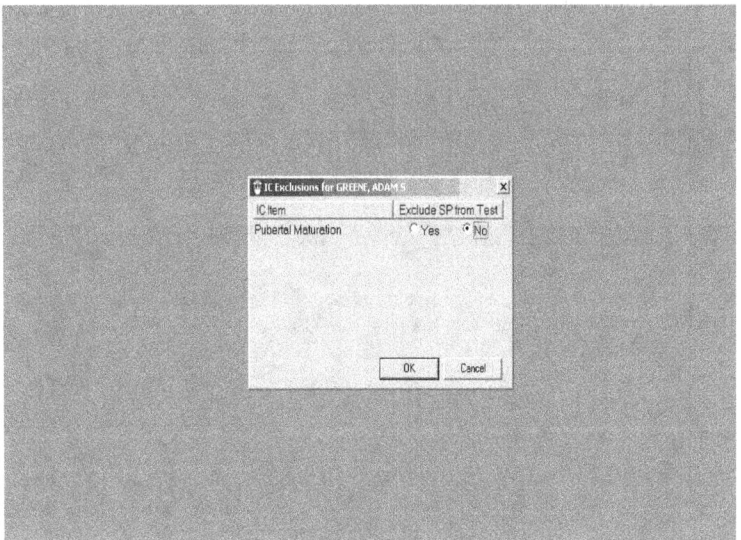

3.6 The Physician's Role in the HPV Proxy Informed Consent

The physician's role in supporting the HPV component of the Proxy interview is not a direct function of the physician exam protocol, but it is a vital role in enhancing response rates of this interview. The HPV informed consent exclusion is accessed through the physician application, and this section explains the physician's responsibility in supporting the consent process.

The male HPV collection will function nearly identically to the HPV swab collection currently done for females. The existing HPV swab protocol in lab will simply be extended to include males aged14 – 59 years, a screen with talking points will be added to Physician for males aged 14 to 59 years, and the Informed Consent Exclusion/Permission window will be modified to include HPV for males aged 14 to 59 years.

The only new component is the parental consent for children aged 14 to 17 years in the proxy application. This will be handled similarly to the pubertal maturation component. A screen has been added to the proxy application to give the responsible adult the opportunity to opt the child out of the HPV collection. The text in the Physician and Proxy screens will be available in both English and Spanish.

Informed Consent Exclusion/Permission window – This window, currently called the Informed Consent Exclusion window, has been renamed the Informed Consent Exclusion/Permission window to indicate its dual purpose of performing informed consent exclusions as well as indicating that a participant did or did not give permission to perform certain tests. This window is available in the Coordinator, Proxy, Phlebotomy, and Physician applications. It will be modified to make the HPV Swab Permission visible to female and male participants aged 14 to 59 years.

Proxy – A screen with talking points will be added for males and females aged 14 to 17 years that gives the responsible adult the option of agreeing to the swab collection and the opportunity to talk to the Physician if he or she doesn't want to opt in. The screen will also enable the person to indicate that the child does not have a responsible adult present, which opts him or her out of the test automatically. Once the pilot ends, the female screen will remain in the application.

Informed Consent Exclusion/Permission Window enhancements – The Informed Consent Exclusion/Permission window has been modified to display HPV Swab Permission for primary males aged 14 to 59 years.

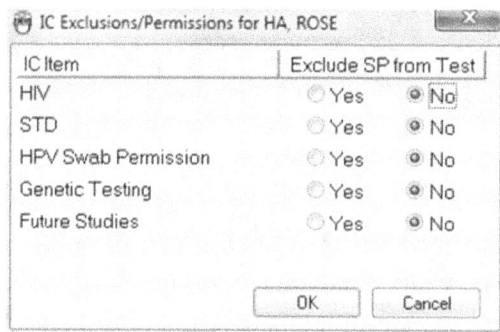

Informed Consent Exclusion/Permission Window

HPV/PM IC Exclusion window – The current informed consent window in Physician has been modified to include the males and females aged 14 to 17 years. This will allow the Physician to un-exclude an SP after he or she has talked to the responsible adult. The existing PM IC Exclusion menu will be modified as shown below to be HPV/PM IC Exclusion

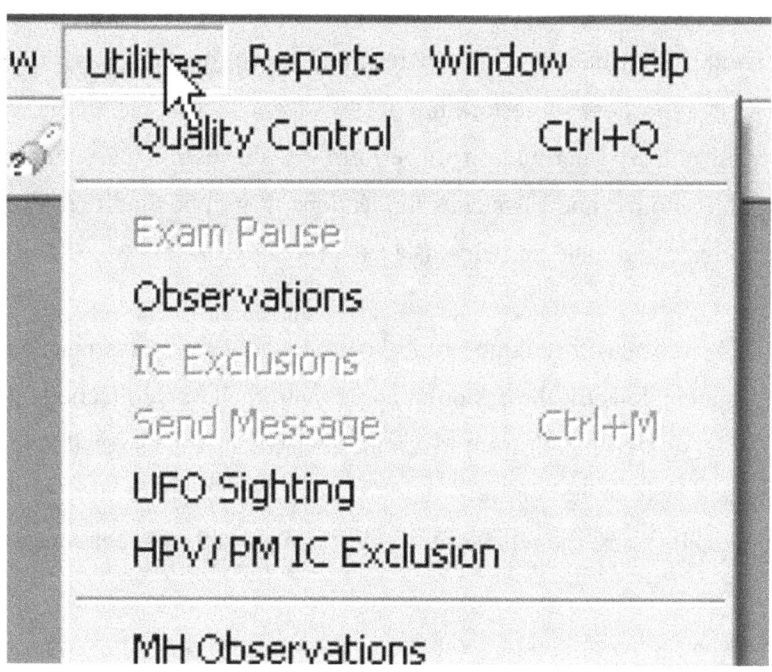

Physician HPV/PM Exclusion Menu Item – Once the Physician selects an SP, the special permission window that displays only Pubertal Maturation will be display. This window has been modified to include HPV swab for both males and females aged 14 to 17 years.

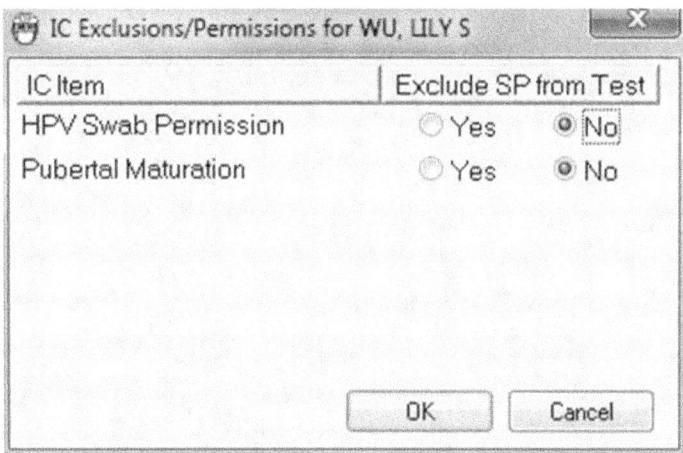

PM/HPV Permission Window in Physician – The proxy application has a slide added for primary males and females aged 14 to 17 years that enables their responsible adult to exclude the SP from getting the HPV swab. This screen will function the same as the pubertal maturation screen.

The following screen has been added, providing information on swab collection.

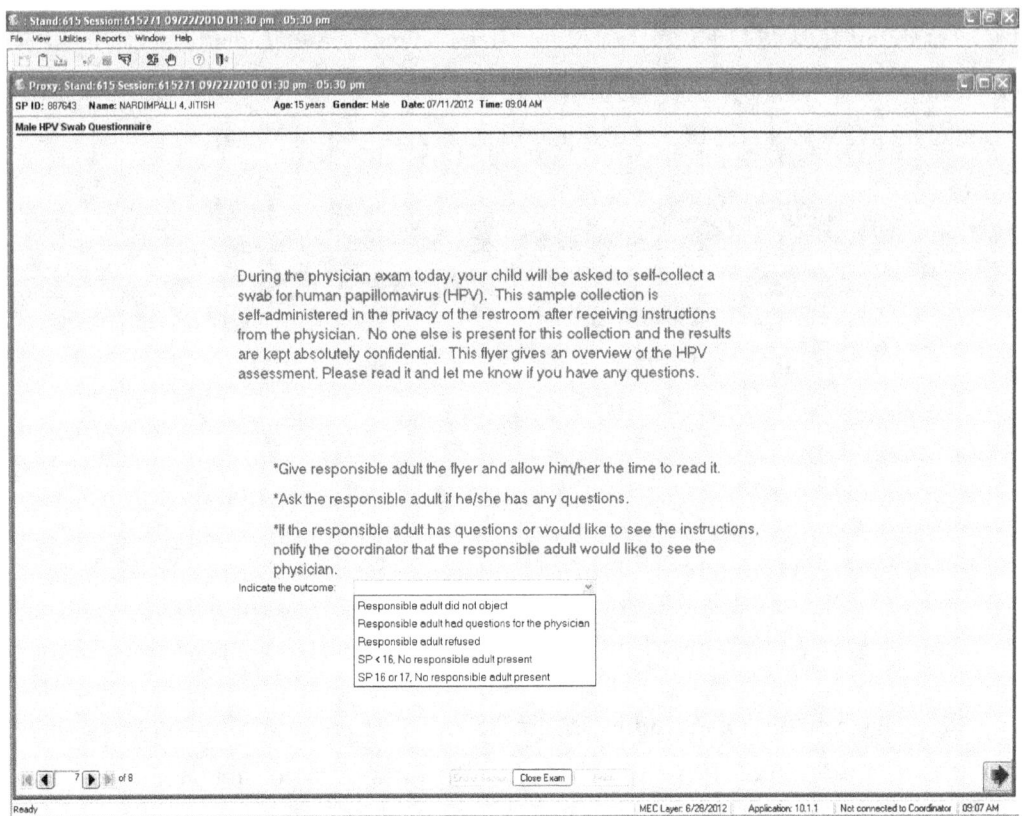

As shown above, there is a drop-down list to indicate the outcome. If the user selects an option other than "reasonable adult did not object" or "SP 16 or 17, no responsible adult present," the application will present the following popup.

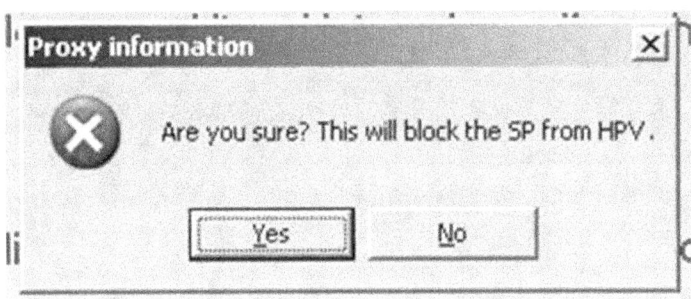

Exclusion Confirmation Message Box

If the user selects Yes, the application will indicate in the Informed Consent Exclusion/Permission module that the SP is excluded from HPV.

Coordination Enhancements

Parental flyers specific to the male and female HPV collection are copied in blue (boys) and pink (girls). Whomever does the proxy will need to use the appropriate color flyer.

If, in the Proxy interview, a parent indicates that he or she wants the 14-17 year old excluded from HPV testing, the MEC interviewers will refer the parent to the physician for final confirmation of that decision. The physician should explain the purpose of the testing once again, ask questions and probe the reasons why the parent is refusing, and try to gain cooperation for the SP's participation in this testing.

If the physician is successful in convincing the parent to allow HPV testing of the child, the IC Exclusions/Permission radio button should be changed to reflect that the SP should not be excluded from the HPV testing.

3.7   The Physician Examination Application and Utilities

3.7.1   Review Functionalities

The Review menu allows the user to access four functions: (1) Referral Review; (2) SP History; (3) Review Other Sessions; and (4) Physician Lookup. The SP History review functionality of the physician application is described in this section. The Referral Review function, Review Other Sessions, and Physician Lookup functionalities are described fully in Chapter 4, as these options are specific to the referral review procedures.

3.7.2   SP History

Medical conditions and medications reported during the home interview for all SPs in the session can be reviewed in the physician's examination under "SP History" (Exhibit 3-45).

- To access "SP History," select "Review" from the toolbar and then choose "SP History."

■ The "SP History" box is displayed (Exhibit 3-45).

Exhibit 3-45. Review menu to select SP History

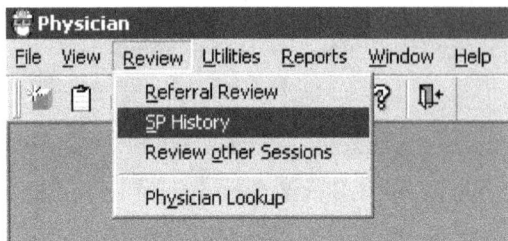

■ A drop-down menu will appear to access individual SP information from the current session only.

■ Two tabs appear on the screen - SP Medical Conditions and Prescriptions. Medical conditions include self-reported illnesses and pregnancy status. The Medications tab displays only medications that were reported during the home interview (Exhibit 3-46).

Exhibit 3-46. SP History screen

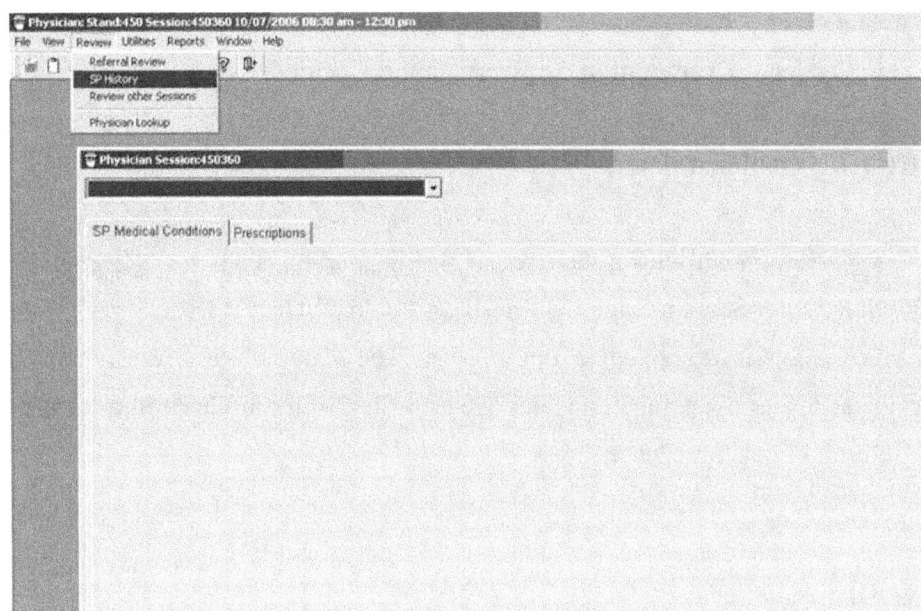

- Each SP's ID number, name, age, and gender are displayed (Exhibit 3-47).

Exhibit 3-47. SP History drop-down menu to select SP from current session

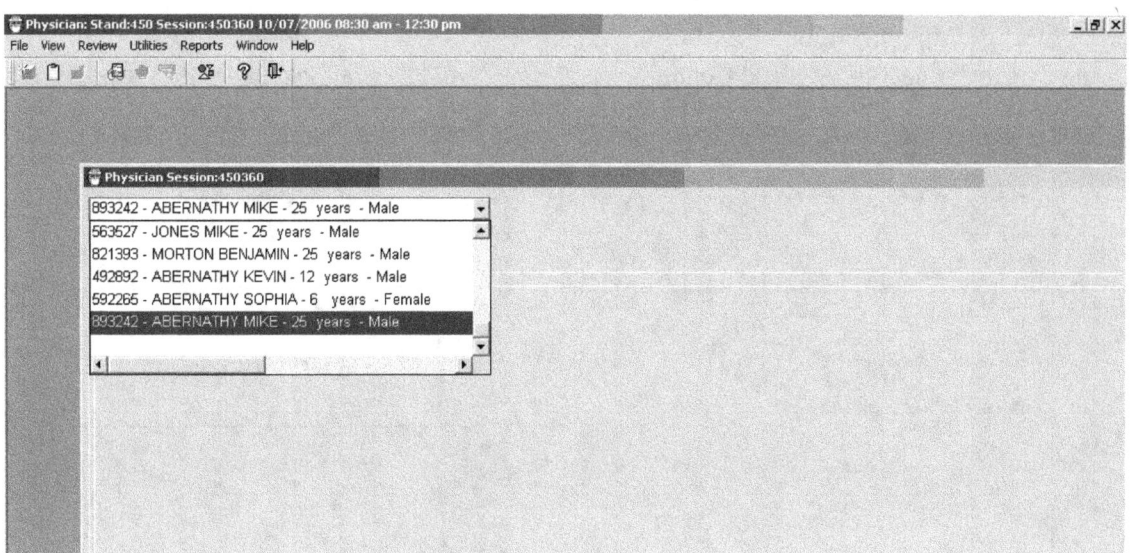

- Highlight the name of the SP to view the medical conditions, medications, and self-reported pregnancy history.

- Switch between the tabs to review medications and medical conditions.

- If no medications or medical conditions have been reported, the screens will indicate this to alert the user that the application is functional and that the screen is blank because nothing was reported during the interview.

Exhibits 3-48 and 3-49 show that no data are available under SP Medical Conditions and Prescriptions tabs.

Exhibit 3-48.
No data available under SP Medical Conditions tab

Exhibit 3-49.
No data available under Prescriptions tab

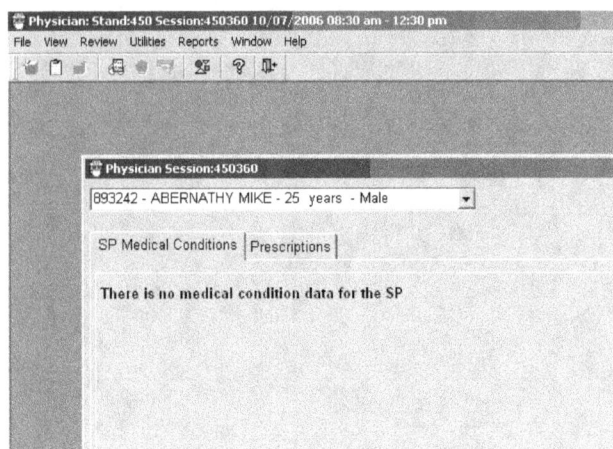 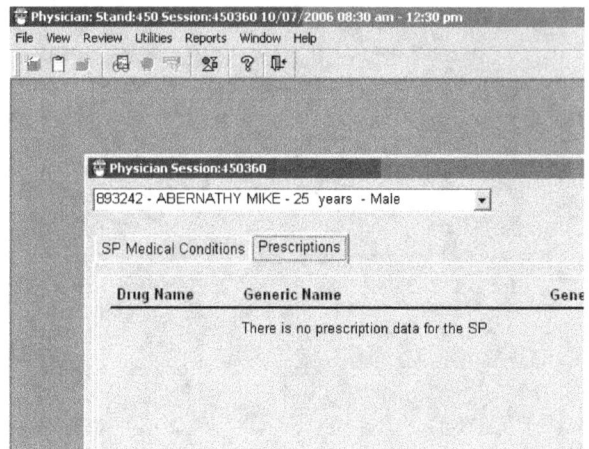

Exhibit 3-50 illustrates the appearance of numerous medical conditions, and Exhibit 3-51 illustrates the appearance of reported medications.

Exhibit 3-50. SP History medical data appearance

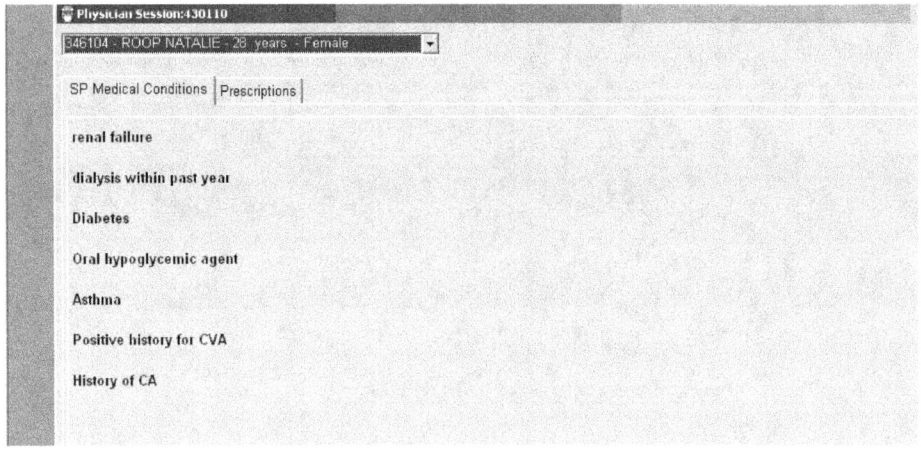

Exhibit 3-51. SP History reported medications appearance

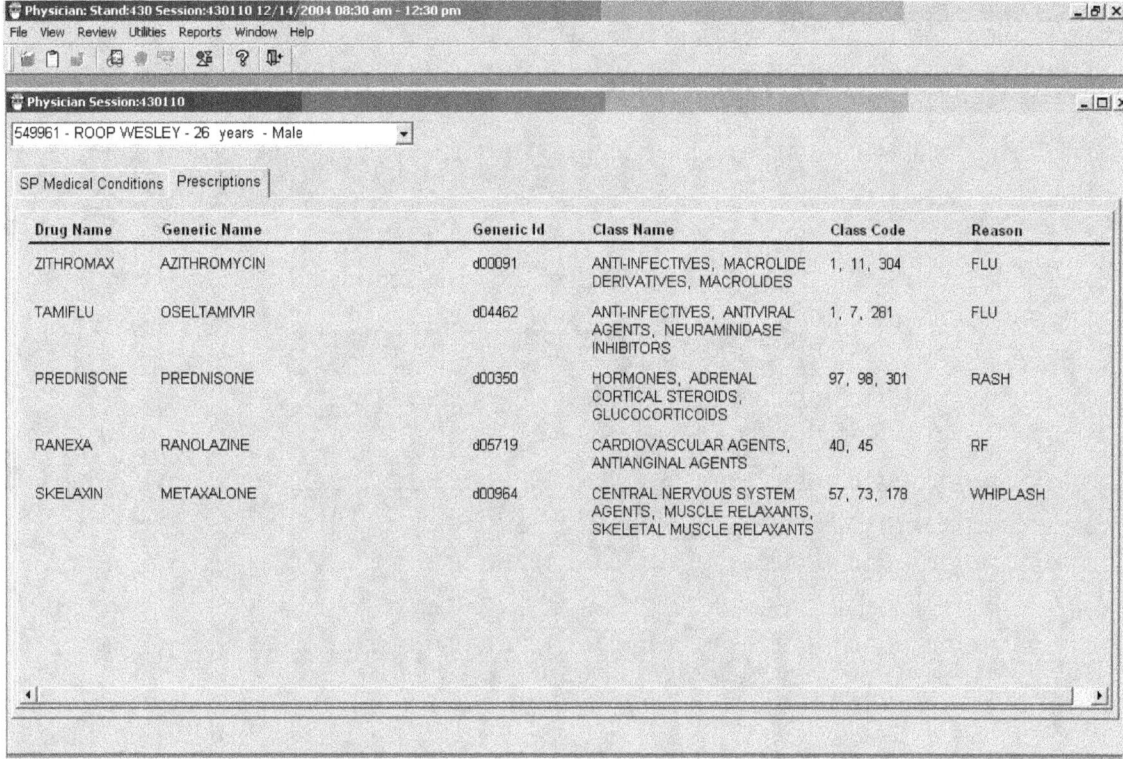

Remember that the field interviewers who gather this information record only the medication information provided by the SP and the indication for the medication as the SP understands it. Therefore, if the physician observes a medication and has any further questions about it, he or she may ask the SP during the physician exam.

3.7.3   Utilities Menu

The utilities menu (Exhibit 3-52) consists of:

- Exam Pause (This functionality is also present on the icon toolbar below the menus.)

- Observations

- IC Exclusions

- Send Message

- UFO Sighting

- MH Observations

- New Emergency Form

- Edit Emergency Form

- English

- Spanish

Exhibit 3-52. Utilities drop-down menu

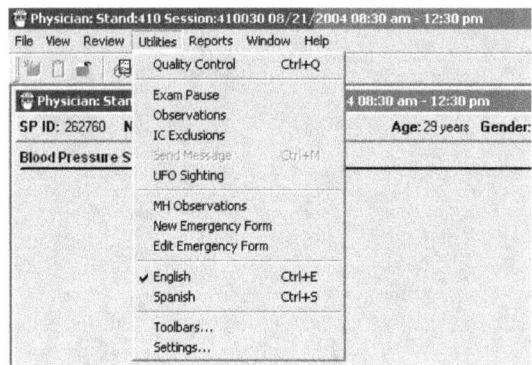

Quality Control

This option opens the quality control dialog box to initiate quality control procedures. See Chapter 7 for quality control procedures.

Exam Pause

This pauses the exam temporarily to stop the exam timer; when the user selects this, a message to the coordinator is sent (exam paused). This should be used if there is an emergency in the MEC.

Observation

The observation field allows the user to document any additional information that could inform the data collection process. See Chapter 7.

IC (Informed Consent) Exclusions

The status of SP informed consent for HIV, STD, HPV, Genetic Testing, and Future Studies is displayed in the box for IC items. The physician can change the status either way if the SP changes his or her mind about these lab tests at any time during the SP's visit to the MEC. For specific guidance on the IC exclusion procedure, see Section 3.4.4.

Send Message

This function allows the physician to send a message to the coordinator.

UFO Sighting

This feature allows the user to document any unusual occurrence that is observed during the operation of a stand. All MEC staff use the UFO utility to document issues relating to: equipment, software, protocols, SPs, trailer facility, supplies, and inventory.

Pubertal Maturation Informed Consent

MH (Mental Health) Observation

See Chapter 4 for specific guidance related to documenting MH observations and referrals.

New Emergency Form

Select this utility when documenting a new Incident/Emergency Form. Refer to Chapter 5.

Edit Emergency Form

Additional or followup information may be added to an existing Incident/Emergency Form using this utility.

English/Spanish

The default setting for language is English, but this utility allows the user to switch between English and Spanish. The physician, when using an interpreter for a Spanish speaking SP, will switch the application to Spanish for the interpreter's benefit (Exhibit 3-53).

Exhibit 3-53. Spanish screen: Example – Shared Exclusion questions

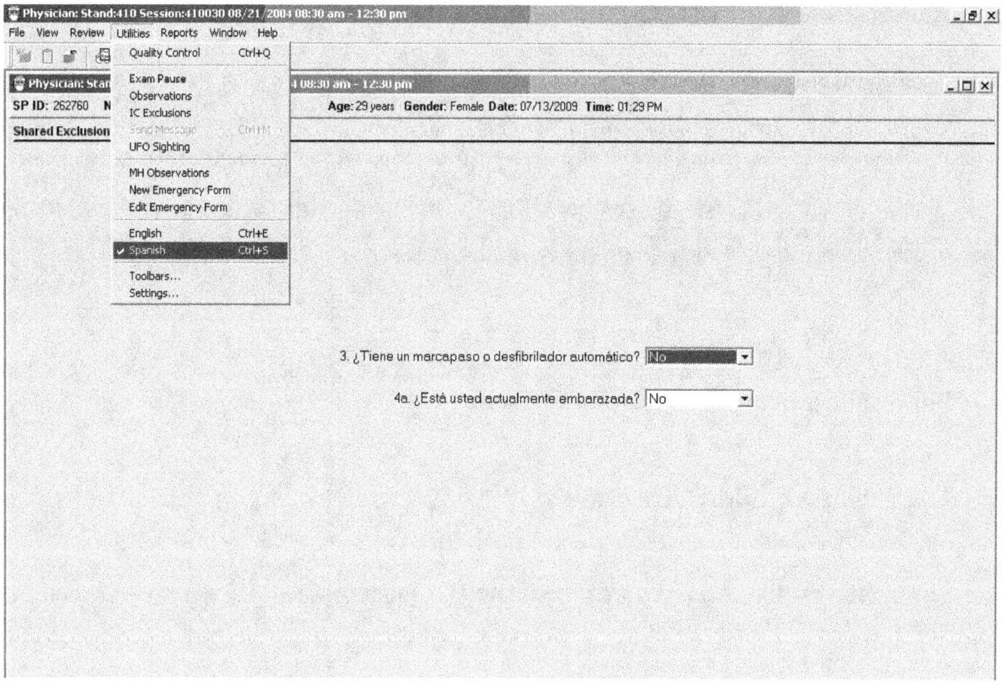

3.8   Report Utility

The Reports utility displays three different reports: (1) The Room Log, (2) Session Preview, and (3) SP Exams (Exhibit 3-54).

Room Log

Exhibit 3-54. Menu for selecting Room Log

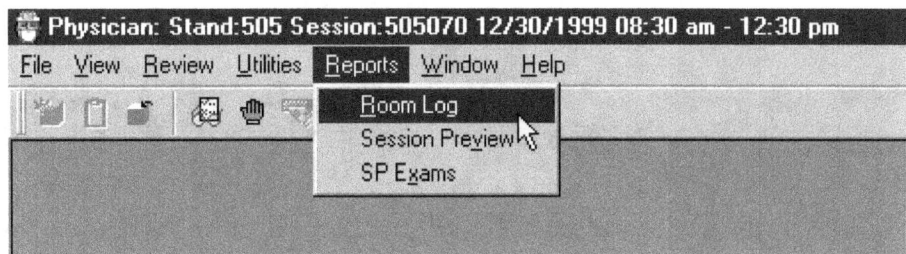

The physician application tracks the status of the examinations and displays the information under the physician room log (Exhibit 3-55).

Exhibit 3-55. The Physician Room Log

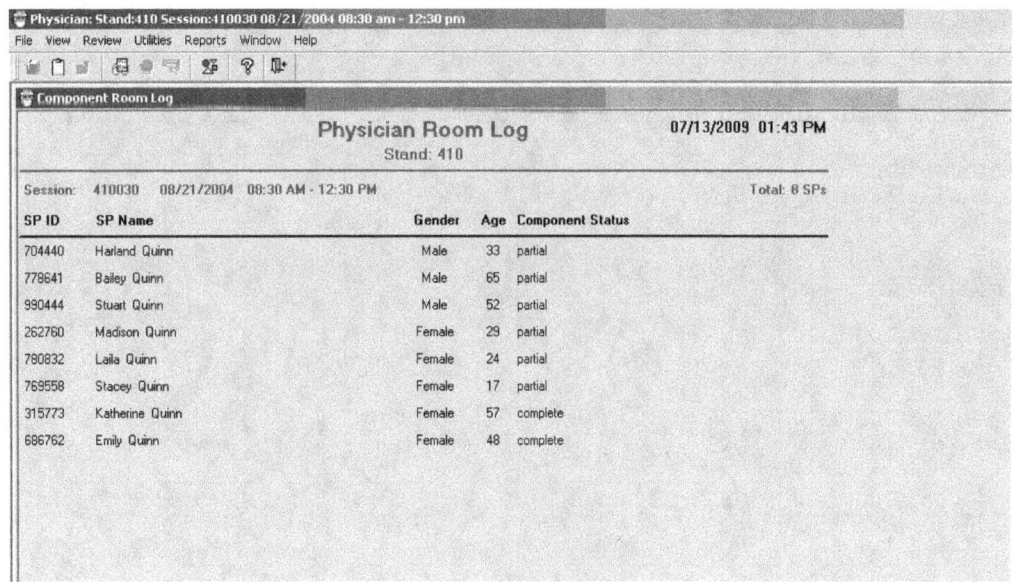

- The room log displays a list of the SPs who are eligible for this examination. All SPs are eligible for the physician's examination. The SP examination status report displays all SPs in the session along with the status and status comment.

- Choose "Reports" from the toolbar and select "Room Log."

Session Preview

- To preview a list of SPs in the current session, select "Reports" from the toolbar.

- Select "Session Preview." (Exhibit 3-56).

Exhibit 3-56. Session preview

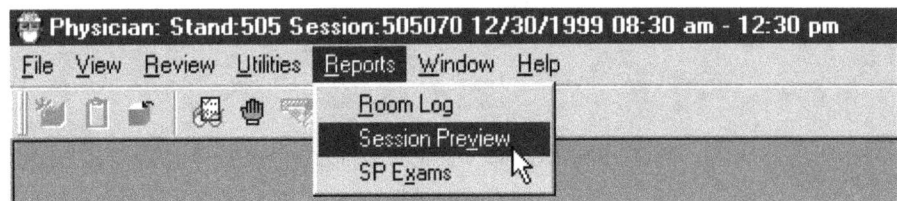

Exhibit 3-57. Session Preview Report

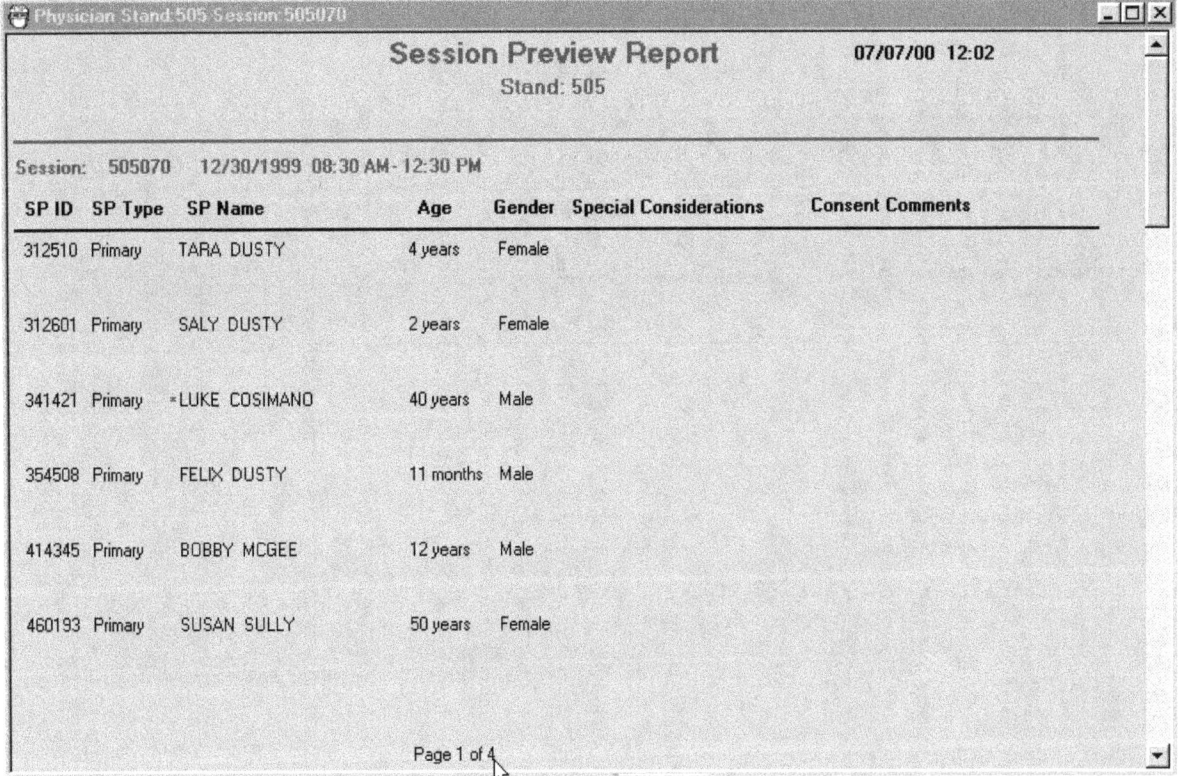

3.8.1   SP Examinations

- To preview the status of the SP examinations in the current session, select "Reports" from the toolbar.

- Select "SP Exams" from the menu (Exhibit 3-58).

Exhibit 3-58. SP examination

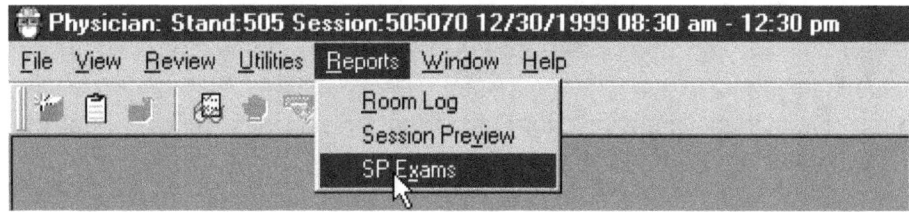

- The SP examination status report can be viewed for each SP in the session.

- The first column lists the components for which the SP is eligible.

- The second column displays the examination status: complete, partial, not done.

- The status remains blank until the SP has been to that component.

- If applicable, the status comment and "Other" comment are also listed.

- Scroll up and down to view all SPs in the session. You can also use age up and page down.

3.8.2   End of Section

■   The "End of Section" button is used to advance to the end of the current section without entering data in the required fields (Exhibit 3-59).

Exhibit 3-59. End of section

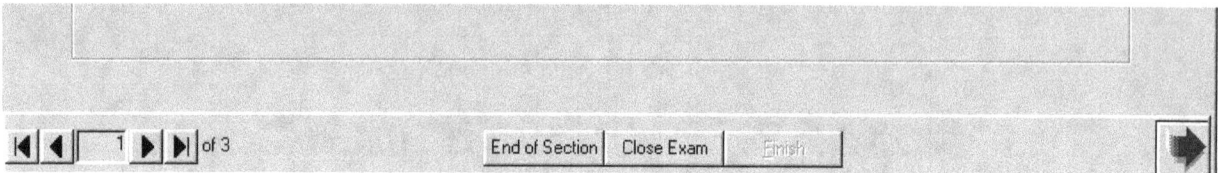

■   The status defaults to "Not Done" and a comment is required. Select the appropriate comment for the situation.

■   One potential situation occurs when there is not enough time at the end of a session to complete the entire examination, but the SP needs the STD and HIV information sheet to be able to obtain test results. The physician opens the examination, selects "End of Section" for the blood pressure and CV exclusion questions. The appropriate comment for both sections is "No Time."

■   The "End of Section" button can be selected from each section. This allows the screens to advance through each section until the STD and HIV results screen appears.

3.8.3   Close Examination Button

■   The correct method of closing an examination is to select the "Finish" button after all the data have been entered.

■   If there is a need to end the examination prematurely, the "Close" button can be selected at the bottom of the screen next to the "End of Section" button.

■   When the "Close" button is selected, a pop-up box is displayed. The examination status defaults to "Not Done" or "Partial" depending on the stage of the examination when the "Close" button was pressed.

■   Select the appropriate comment from the drop-down list (Exhibit 3-60).

Exhibit 3-60. Prematurely closing examination

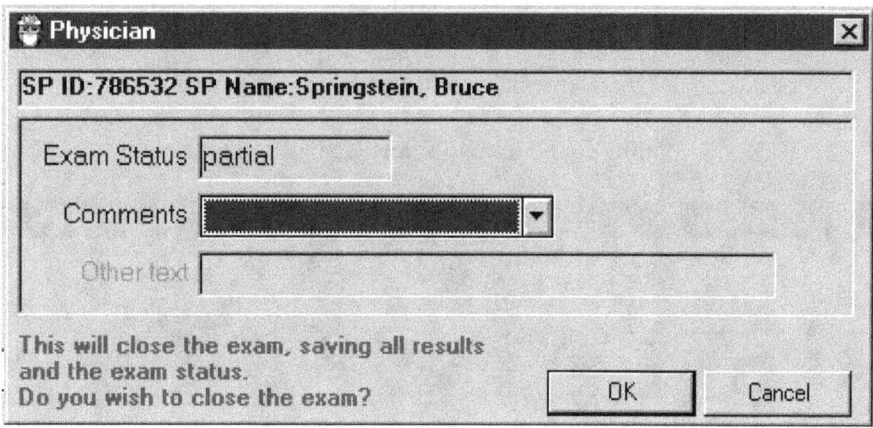

3.8.4   Pausing an Examination

■   There may be situations where the physician is needed in another room in the MEC. If this occurs during an examination, select the icon with the red hand (the Pause icon).

■   Clicking this icon pauses the examination in the physician's room. The timer for the examination stops (Exhibit 3-61).

Exhibit 3-61. Pause an examination

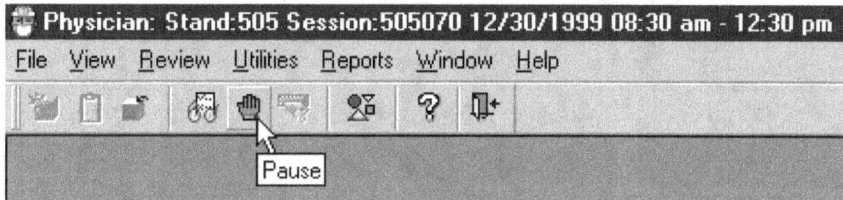

■   The Pause icon acts as a toggle and the timer will not start again until the icon is clicked again.

■   Examination pause may also be accessed from selecting "Utilities" from the Toolbar and then selecting "Examination Pause" from the menu.

OMB Statement

■ The OMB statement is found under the Help menu on the toolbar. Choose "Help," and then select OMB statement from the menu (Exhibit 3-62).

Exhibit 3-62 Menu to select OMB statement

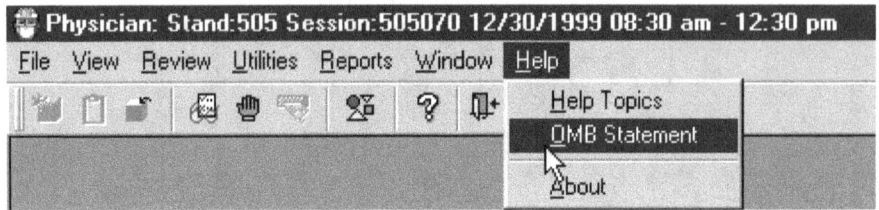

Exhibit 3-63. OMB statement

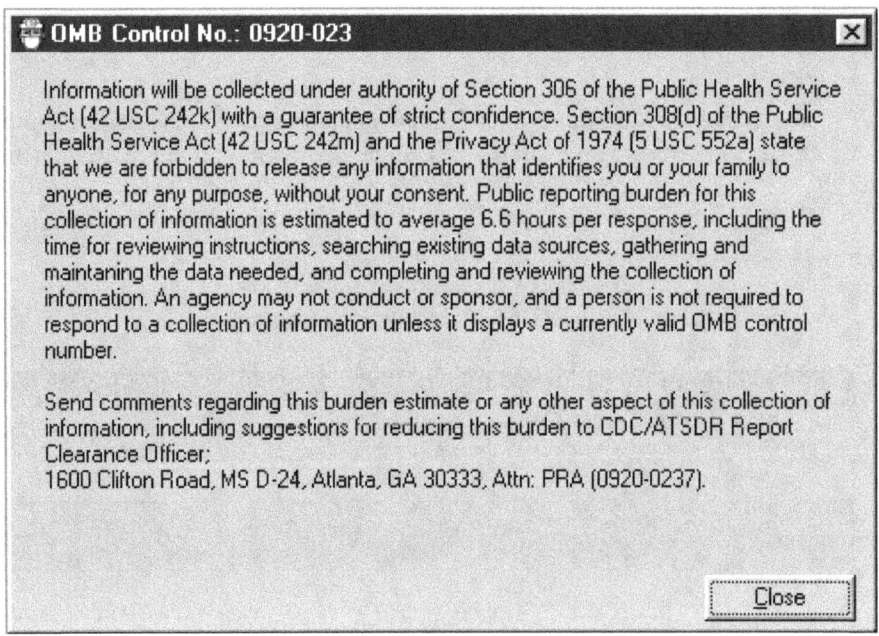

4. REFERRALS

4.1   Medical Referrals

Although the primary purpose of the MEC examination is data collection, not diagnosis or treatment, the examination may produce findings that warrant further medical attention. There is an obligation to inform SPs of any abnormal results from the examinations and to refer SPs to appropriate providers for treatment. MEC physicians are responsible for referrals. Each examination component has a referral process built into the ISIS system. This automatic process alerts examining physicians to findings that may require a referral. SPs and their providers may already be aware of some findings, but others may have been revealed for the first time during the MEC exam. MEC physicians review the data provided and the categories set forth by the Physicians Advisory Group (PAG) to determine what type of referral, if any, is needed.

MEC physicians can arrange for a referral to a care provider for SPs who do not have a local provider. The local providers agree to accept referrals from the MEC examination prior to the arrival of the mobile examination team and prior to any examinations being carried out in the MEC. These advance arrangements are made through an advance arrangement team that includes a physician from the National Center for Health Statistics.

Referrals may be based on data collected during MEC examination components (examination data-related referrals) or based on subjective or objective observations made by any MEC examiner (observation referrals). These two types of referrals are described in detail in this section.

Examination data-related referrals are based on predefined criterion levels from the examination data. These criterion levels were defined by the physician advisory group and are built into the ISIS system so that when the limits are exceeded, the system automatically flags this information to the physician for the specific SP. The flag occurs when component data that are above or below the predefined limits are recorded. The examination components that send data-related referrals to the physician system are the laboratory (pregnancy and complete blood count), mental health (from the MEC Interviewer health examination), blood pressure from the physician's examination, and spirometry results.

This chapter describes the referral procedures for exam-specific data results, as well as independent observations:

- Laboratory data: CBC and Pregnancy Tests;

- Blood Pressure;

- General Observations;

- Mental Health;

- Cognitive Functioning; and

- Automated Referral Procedures in the Physician Application.

4.2   Referral Levels

The MEC physician examiner makes decisions about referring SPs for additional care based on a system rated by three levels (Exhibit 4-1). This is important, because different MEC examinations generate various categories of urgent information that are often different, one from the other. Findings that are outside the normal limits should be reviewed by a qualified medical professional to determine if additional followup care is needed. These three levels of referral apply across all MEC examinations. The Physician's Advisory Group (PAG) at the National Center for Health Statistics (NCHS) defined the action required for each referral level. The edit limits or ranges for referrals in each component were defined by the component specialists and consultants and subsequently reviewed and approved by the PAG. Based on the results of any component of the MEC examination, physicians place SPs in one of three referral categories. They provide guidance to the MEC physician regarding the urgency of an examination finding. The highest, most urgent referral is a Level 1 referral. Level 3 represents an examination finding that the physician reviews, but does not refer the SP for further care. This method of referral assures that physicians from both exam teams review all findings that appear out of the standardized norm, and that there is a record made that the physician reviewed the findings and made an informed decision, based from their medical background, about whether the SP should be referred.

Table 4-1.   Table of referral levels

Referral level	Category	Action
1	4	Indicates major medical findings that warrant immediate attention by a health care provider.
2	3	Indicates major medical findings that warrant attention by a health care provider within the next 2 weeks. These findings are expected to cause adverse effects within this time period and they have previously been undiagnosed, unattended, nonmanifested, or not communicated to the examinee by his or her personal health care provider.
3	1 & 2	Indicates no major negative medical findings, or minor medical findings that an examinee already knows about, and is under care for, or findings that do not require prompt attention by a medical provider.

4.2.1   Level 1 Referrals

These referrals are generated when there are major medical findings that warrant immediate attention by a health care provider, such as a dangerously high blood pressure, and life threatening emergencies. SPs determined to need a Level 1 referral usually terminate further MEC examinations. SPs are transferred out of the MEC and into a hospital or other care facility. SPs who refuse treatment from this level of referral are asked to sign a release stating that they are aware of the examination findings, but they are refusing treatment against the advice of the MEC physician. SPs must sign the release form before leaving the MEC. The release is available in both English and Spanish.

4.2.2   Level 2 Referrals

The MEC physician generates these referrals when there are major medical findings that require attention by a health care provider in the next 2 weeks because they are expected to cause adverse effects within this time. Level 2 referrals allow SPs to continue MEC examinations; however, they are advised to see their primary care provider within 2 weeks following the examination. A high, but not dangerously high blood pressure is an example of a Level 2 referral.

4.2.3 Level 3 Referrals

Level 3 referrals consist of either no out-of-range medical findings or minor medical findings that an examinee already knows about, is under care for, or does not require prompt attention by a medical provider. Level 3 findings do not necessarily generate referrals. Examinees receive a report of the findings from many of the examination components before leaving the MEC. In addition, a detailed Report of Findings is sent from NCHS approximately 2 to 4 months after completion of the examination. The latter report contains the results of some findings that are not available before SPs leave the MEC.

4.3 Laboratory Referrals

Urine and blood are collected for various laboratory tests on all SPs ages 1 year and older. A complete and detailed description of these tests can be found in the *NHANES Laboratory Procedures Manual*. Two laboratory findings are given to the participant in the preliminary Report of Findings prior to SPs leaving the mobile examination center—the complete blood count and the urine pregnancy test. When these findings are outside the predetermined criterion levels for referral, physicians decide whether a referral is needed. When a referral is indicated, the physician provides the information to the SP. The laboratory findings and the parameters that generate referral advice to the physician are shown in Tables 4-2 and 4-3 on page 4-10. The two laboratory results reviewed by the physician are the urine pregnancy test and the complete blood count.

4.3.1 Pregnancy Referral Requirements

Urine pregnancy tests are done on all SPs between the ages of 12 through 59 years, and on girls ages 8 through 11 years if they reported menarche during the household interview. The physician is the **only** person who discusses the pregnancy results with the SP since some SPs may be unaware of their pregnancy at the time of the test. The physician discloses results of positive pregnancy tests to the SP, unless the SP is 18 or over and had already reported the pregnancy during the interview. SPs under 18 years of age always see the physician when a positive pregnancy test is reported. Negative pregnancy test results are provided to SPs only upon the SP's specific request. Physicians discuss the importance of prenatal health care in situations where SPs have not seen a health care provider when they have a positive pregnancy test. Referrals are facilitated if appropriate. SPs with no source of prenatal care are referred to a local public health clinic or primary care provider.

4.3.2 Unmarried Minors Pregnancy Referrals

The finding of a positive pregnancy test in an unmarried minor (under age 18) requires physicians to conduct a brief evaluation to determine the level of counseling and referral necessary. The physician discloses a positive pregnancy test result directly to the minor.

Federal law requires physicians to report child abuse. These pregnancy referral requirements are based on child abuse laws for SPs less than 18 years of age. When counseling the pregnant minor, physicians take a brief history to determine whether the pregnancy may have resulted from sexual abuse. The index of suspicion for sexual abuse is based solely on what a minor discloses, rather than a full medical evaluation. Young women may refuse to provide information surrounding their pregnancy. If the information provided by a minor leads the physician to be concerned about possible, probable, or definite sexual abuse, **the parent/guardian is informed** and a report is filed with Child Protective Services (CPS). If the physician is unsure whether to report, the physician discusses the case with a social worker at Child Protective Services. When presenting the case, MEC physicians do not use the minor's name or any other identifier. If the social worker and physician agree that the referral to CPS should be made, the physician may provide the name and address of the minor. Physicians may follow up the verbal reporting with a written documentation of findings relevant to the reporting. **These written reports are private, and are not collected in the NHANES database.**

If the minor is under 14 years of age, physicians discuss the circumstances of the pregnancy with the child, inform the parent, and report the case to Child Protective Services (CPS). Pregnancy in such a young age is probable child abuse. If the physician is informed that the child is already receiving prenatal care, the physician verifies this information directly with the provider. In cases where the child is already receiving prenatal care and has received a full medical evaluation, no report to CPS is indicated.

If the minor is 14 years and older, physicians disclose results directly to the minor and assesses (a) whether the minor is already receiving prenatal care or pregnancy counseling, (b) whether minor's parent/guardian is aware of the pregnancy, and (c) whether the pregnancy is a result of child sexual abuse. If a minor who is 14 years or older is already receiving prenatal health care, physicians confirm this with the local provider. No further referral or parental notification is necessary unless other examination findings meet the criteria for referral. If the minor is not receiving prenatal care, the physician discusses the importance of a medical evaluation and pregnancy counseling for the SP, and facilitates a referral. SPs with no source of care are referred to a local public health clinic or primary care provider. Because a parent/guardian should be informed of a minor's pregnancy if she is not receiving prenatal care, the physician will offer to help the minor tell her parent/guardian before leaving the MEC. **If the minor strongly opposes the disclosure of the pregnancy test results to a parent or guardian, the physician respects the minor's confidentiality.**

4.3.3   Complete Blood Count

The MEC physician reviews and interprets all CBC results. Abnormal results constituting action limits flash and transmit to the physician immediately. The physician determines if referral for the SP for treatment is necessary. The medical technologist sends an observation to the physician whenever a critical or action limit is detected for any CBC parameter. This observation includes the date, time, responsible laboratory individual, person notified, and test results.

A new hematology analyzer (Coulter DXH 800) is replacing the existing analyzer in all three mobile examination centers. Once installed and tested, the Complete Blood Count section of the NHANES Report of Findings will be based on the new Coulter DXH 800. This machine is more sophisticated and additional parameters will be reported.

This machine directly measures the red blood count (RBC), white blood count (WBC), hemoglobin (Hg), and differential percentage. The mean corpuscular volume (MCV), red cell distribution (RDW), platelets (PLT), and mean platelet volume (MPV) are derived from histograms while other values are calculated. Reference ranges for normal values (Tables 4-2 and 4-3) were calculated from NHANES data, last updated in 2003. The following values are transmitted to the physician for review:

1.   **Red Blood Count** – Elevated RBC may reflect primary polycythemia (polycythemia rubra vera) or secondary causes of polycythemia (stress erythrocytosis, diseases associated with low oxygen, certain renal disorders, etc.). Decreased RBC count may indicate anemia.

2.   **Hemoglobin** – Abnormal Hgb measurements usually reflect the same conditions as the RBC count and can define the type of anemia.

Table 4-2.   Complete Blood Count Reference Ranges—Males

Age in years	1-5		6-18		19-65		66+	
White blood cell count (SI)	4.3	14.6	3.6	11.5	3.9	11.8	3.8	12.1
Red cell count (SI)	3.98	5.3	4.14	5.78	4.18	5.86	3.57	5.67
Hemoglobin (g/dL)	10.7	14.2	11.9	16.9	13.1	17.5	11.4	17.1
Hematocrit (%)	32.1	41.7	35.3	49.9	38.7	51.4	33.9	50.9
Mean cell volume (fL)	68.2	88.8	75.6	94.6	79.8	99.1	81.4	102.7
Mean cell hemoglobin (pg)	22.3	30.6	25	32.3	26.3	34	26.3	35
MCHC (g/dL)	32.3	35.6	32.3	35.3	32.3	35.3	32.1	35.1
Red cell distribution width (%)	11.4	15.8	11.4	14	11.4	14.5	11.8	16.2
Platelet count (%) SI	212	546	179	439	152	386	124	384
Mean platelet volume (fL)	6.1	8.9	6.6	10	6.8	10.1	6.6	10.2
Lymphocyte percent (%)	22.8	68.4	17.5	54.3	16.1	47.9	12.3	46.4
Monocyte percent (%)	4.6	15.2	4.8	13.7	4.4	13.5	4.6	14
Segmented neutrophils percent (%)	17.6	67.1	30.3	72.8	37.8	74.6	39.5	78.1
Eosinophils percent (%)	0.7	11.3	0.7	11.5	0.7	8.5	0.6	8.8
Basophils percent (%)	0.1	2.5	0.1	1.6	0.1	1.6	0.1	1.6

Table 4-3.   Complete Blood Count Reference Ranges—Females

Age in years	1-5		6-18		19-65		66+	
White blood cell count (SI)	4.3	14	3.9	12.2	4.1	12.9	4	11.6
Red cell count (SI)	3.96	5.28	3.84	5.24	3.64	5.2	3.51	5.34
Hemoglobin (g/dL)	11	14.2	11.2	15.1	10.6	15.6	10.9	15.9
Hematocrit (%)	32.5	41.9	33.5	44.6	32	45.9	32.8	47
Mean cell volume (fL)	70.2	89.1	74.7	94.9	74.6	98.2	80.3	100.6
Mean cell hemoglobin (pg)	23.3	30.8	24.5	32.6	24.3	33.8	26.4	34.5
MCHC (g/dL)	32.4	35.5	32.3	35.3	32.1	35.3	32.3	35.1
Red cell distribution width (%)	11.3	15.4	11.3	14.8	11.4	16.3	11.6	16.3
Platelet count (%) SI	215	547	190	446	168	441	155	428
Mean platelet volume (fL)	6.1	8.9	6.6	10	6.8	10.2	6.7	10.5
Lymphocyte percent (%)	21.6	68.8	17.2	54.7	14.1	47.6	13.7	46.9
Monocyte percent (%)	4.2	14.4	4.3	12.7	3.8	11.6	4.4	12.8
Segmented neutrophils percent (%)	19.4	69.5	31.9	74.3	39.8	78.1	40.9	78.1
Eosinophils percent (%)	0.6	9.9	0.6	9.9	0.6	7.3	0.6	7.5
Basophils percent (%)	0.1	2.5	0.1	1.6	0.1	1.7	0.1	1.7

3. **Hematocrit** – Abnormal hematocrit values usually reflect the same conditions as the RBC and can help define the type of anemia.

4. **White Blood Count** – High values (leukocytosis) may indicate a primary condition such as leukemia or a secondary condition such as infection. Low values (leukopenia) may indicate the presence of autoimmune, neoplastic, drug-induced, congenital, or other conditions. See below.

5. **Lymphocytes** – Elevated counts (lymphocytosis) may be primary (leukemias, lymphomas, monoclonal B cell lymphocytosis) or secondary (viral infection, acute physical stress, pertussis, and chronic disorders such as autoimmune disease and cancer). Depressed counts (lymphopenia) can reflect a variety of uncommon inherited disorders or the more frequent acquired conditions such as viral and certain bacterial infections, the effects of immunosupressive agents, and some chronic diseases.

6. **Monocytes** – These cells, derived from the bone marrow are the precursors of tissue macrophages. Monocytosis is often seen in chronic infections (TB, brucellosis), acute protozoan and rickettsial diseases, and in neutropenia. Uncommon malignant disorders (monocytic leukemia, histiocytic lymphoma) and nonmalignant conditions (hemophagocytic syndromes) can also cause it.

7. **Neutrophils** – Elevated neutrophils (granulocytosis) are seen in both primary (myelocytic leukemias, polycythemia rubra vera) and, more commonly, in secondary conditions (bacterial infections, chronic inflammation, corticosteroid use, cigarette smoking, etc.). Hereditary neutrophilia is rare. Decreased neutrophils (leukopenia) can also result from primary (myeloid malignancies, congenital disorders) and secondary (drug effect, viral infection, splenomegaly, autoimmune, and hereditary disorders) conditions.

8. **MCH** – The mean corpuscular hemoglobin, in picograms, is calculated from the ratio of Hgb to RBC. This measure of hemoglobin per RBC is used in conjunction with the MCV and the MCHC to further define anemias. For example, the MCH is elevated in macrocytic anemias and depressed in microcytic, hypochromic anemia.

9. **MCHC** – The mean corpuscular hemoglobin concentration is derived from the ratio of the Hgb to the VPRC. It is also used to help define anemias, being elevated in macrocytic anemias and depressed in hypochromic anemias.

10. **RDW** – The red cell distribution width is a measure of the homogeniety of the RBC population. It is analogous to anisocytosis seen on microscopic examination. Most macrocytic and microcytic anemias, especially with reticulocytosis, will cause an increased RDW. There is no known pathological cause of a decreased RDW.

11. **Platelets** – A decreased platelet count (thrombocytopenia) can be caused by production abnormalities (radiation, drug-induced, cancer, folate or B12 deficiency, myelodysplasia syndromes, HIV, alcohol abuse, etc.), accelerated removal (ITP, SLE, rug antibodies, certain infections, etc.), and hypersplenism. Elevated counts (thrombocytosis) can be primary (myeloproliferative disorders such as CML and PRV, essential thrombocythemia) or secondary (acute trauma, chronic iron deficiency, inflammatory disease, cancer, splenectomy, etc.).

The machine might produce "suspect" messages – i.e., sickled cells, left shift, and giant platelets. If there is a suspect message (see table below), the message for the NHANES ROF (see right column below) will be printed on the bottom of the Complete Blood Count report with the statement, "This finding was not confirmed by microscopy and followup may be necessary." The MEC physician reviews all the Complete Blood Count results while the participant is still in the examining center. If a referral is necessary, the physician will complete a referral form.

Suspect message	ID	Message for NHANES ROF
Dimorphic Reds	1262	At least two populations of red blood cells may be present.
Giant Platelets	1263	Giant platelets may be present.
Imm Grans	1264	The following cells may be present: a) metamyelocytes and myelocytes and/or promyelocytes, or b) myelocytes and/or promyelocytes without metamyeloctytes.
Left Shift	1265	A left shift may be present. The specimen may contain metamyelocytes without myelocytes, promyelocytes, or blasts.
LY Blast	1266	Lymphocyte blast cells may be present.
MO Blast	1267	Monocyte blast cells may be present.
NE Blast	1268	Neutrophil blast cells may be present.
RBC Frag/Microcytes	1269	Red blood cell fragments and/or microcytic red blood cells may be present.
Red Cell Agglut	1270	Red blood cells clumps or rouleaux may be present.
Sickled Cells	1271	Sickled red blood cells may be present.
Variant LY	1272	Variant lymphocytes or immature or abnormal lymphocytes may be present.

The CBC review (Exhibit 4-1) tab under referral review will be split into an upper and lower section (as shown below). The upper section will display the information currently sent to this section. The lower section of the page will display the information in the table above. Both sections should have a scrolling capability should there be a large amount of information on either section of the page.

Exhibit 4-1. Referral review for Complete Blood Count

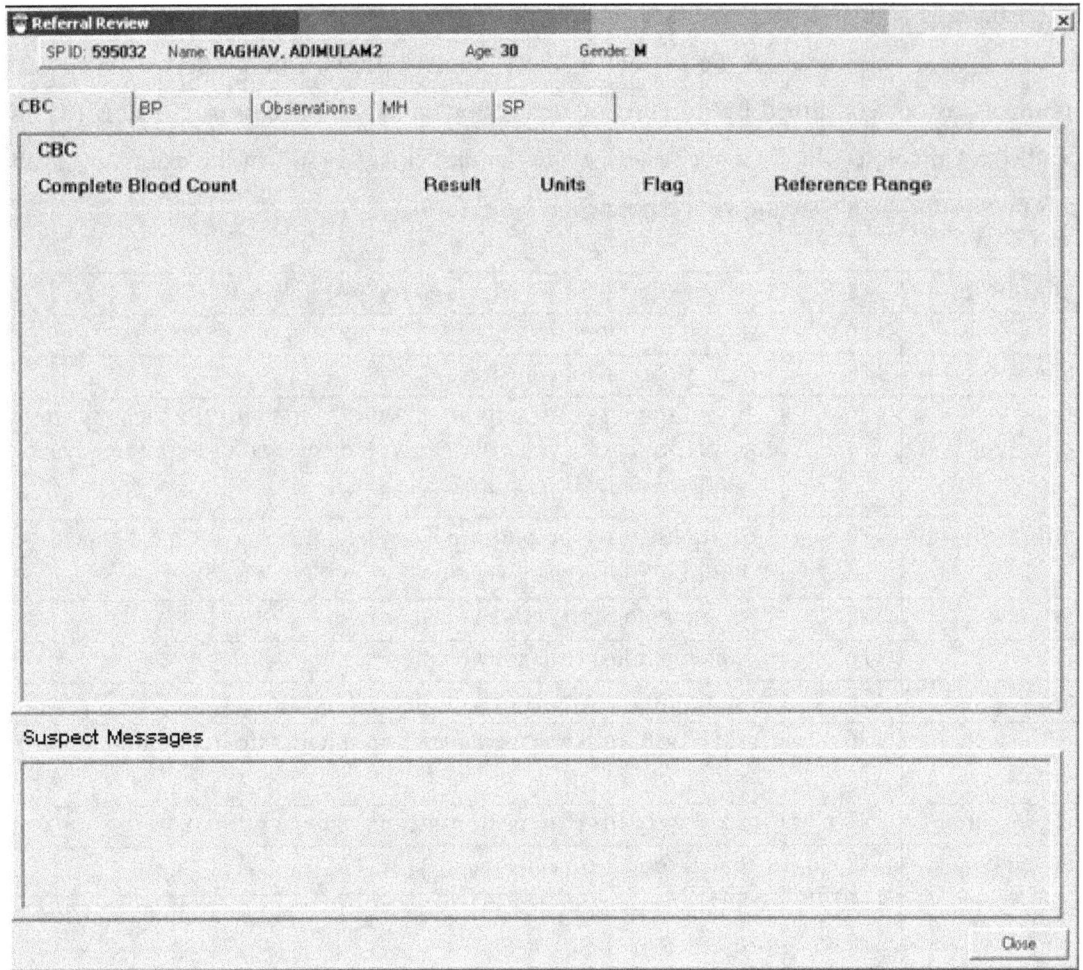

Action Limits. Action limits are a guide to inform the physician that a CBC result(s) is/are abnormal. Since all specimens are run in duplicate, there is no reason to retest the sample in the vast majority of cases.

4.3.3.1 CBC Action Limits

The following limits constitute "Action Limits" where the referral application alerts the physician when present:

- WBC male and female (all ages) $<$ or $=$ to $3 \times 10^3 \, \mu L$ or $>$ or $=$ to $16.0 \times 10^3 \, \mu L$;
- Hgb male and female ($<$6 years) $<$6.5 g/dL or $>$14.5 g/dL;
- Hgb female ($>$6 years) $<$6.5 g/dL or $>$16.0 g/dL;
- Hgb male ($>$6 years) $<$6.5 g/dL or $>$18.0 g/dL; and
- PLT male and female (all ages) $<$50 $\times 10^3 \, \mu L$ or $>$800 $\times 10^3 \, \mu L$.

4.3.3.2 Repeating a CBC

In rare circumstances a result from the complete blood count may be an extreme value that would be considered a "panic" value in clinical practice. An example is severe thrombocytopenia. The physician may repeat the complete blood count if the participant reports no history of nosebleeds or prolonged bleeding and the physician verifies that the site of the first venipuncture clotted normally. The second complete blood count will overwrite the first results in ISIS and will be used for reporting and referrals. Please follow the procedures below when it is determined that a repeat CBC must be drawn.

If the physician feels a repeat blood count is needed, then he or she has the discretion to discuss this with the SP and have the phlebotomist draw a 3-ML EDTA tube for a repeat CBC if the SP agrees. Prior to a second phlebotomy, the physician should visually inspect the site of the first venipuncture to rule out prolonged bleeding. If the puncture site looks normal, then a second phlebotomy can be requested. The SP always has the right to refuse the blood draw. The need for this action should be rare as evidenced by the four total low platelet counts in the last 2 years.

After the physician reviews the findings with the SP, and the SP agrees to a repeat CBC phlebotomy:

- The physician should consult with the MEC manager and chief med tech to arrange to have the blood drawn at the next earliest opportunity.

- If the SP is eligible for the second GTT blood draw, we currently require the phlebotomist to draw any tubes that might not have been collected during the first blood draw. The second 3-mL EDTA tube could be drawn at that time but the phlebotomist will need to be alerted because the tube will not display on the GTT blood draw protocol screen.

- If the SP is not eligible for the GTT blood draw, then he or she will need to be walked to phlebotomy to have the blood drawn.

- This additional blood draw will not be supported by the laboratory and phlebotomy applications.

- As long as the SP has not checked out of the MEC, or if the Report of Findings has **not** been printed, the lab application will allow the med techs to overwrite the existing CBC data with the new data and the new data will become the final result of record.

- The physician will document this event under observations in the physician application.

When the values from the Beckman Coulter® report are interpreted, various interfering substances and conditions may affect these parameters:

- Abnormal BUN, glucose, or sodium levels could affect the MCV.

- Abnormal WBCs could affect lymphocytes, monocytes, and granulocytes.

- Abnormally small WBCs could affect white count, lymphocytes, monocytes, and granulocytes.

- Clumped platelets could affect white count, lymphocytes, monocytes, granulocytes, RBC, MCV, RDW, platelet count, and MPV.

- Cryofibrinogen and cryoglobulin crystals could affect white count, lymphocytes, monocytes, granulocytes, RBC, hemoglobin, platelet count, and MPV.

- An elevated WBC could affect RBC, hemoglobin, MCV, RDW, platelet count, and MPV parameters.

- Fragile WBCs could affect white count, lymphocytes, monocytes, granulocytes, platelet count, and MPV.

- Giant platelets could affect white count, lymphocytes, monocytes, granulocytes, RBC, MCV, RDW, platelet count, and MPV.

- Hemolyzed specimens could affect RBC, hemoglobin, platelet count, and MPV.

- Lipemic specimens could affect MCV.

- Severely icteric plasma causes increased hemoglobin. Evaluate CBC result carefully and report all parameters except the hemoglobin result.

- Nucleated RBC's could affect the white count, lymphocytes, monocytes, granulocytes, and hemoglobin values.

Possible causes of abnormal parameters:

- High RBC, Hgb, or HCT—dehydration, polycythemia, shock, chronic hypoxia;

- Low RBC, Hgb or HCT—anemia, thalassemia and other hemoglobinopathies;

- Low MCV—microcytic anemia;

- High MCV—macrocytic anemia, liver disease;

- Low WBC—sepsis, marrow hypoplasia;

- High WBC—acute stress, infection, malignancies;

- Low platelets—risk of bleeding; and

- High platelets—risk of thrombosis.

4.4 Blood Pressure Referrals

4.4.1 Blood Pressure Referrals – Adults

Tables 4-4 through 4-7 provide the matrix of combinations of systolic and diastolic blood pressure results and the referrals that are generated when these BPs are present for adults. The left column specifies the minimum and maximum systolic pressure groupings. The first row specifies the minimum and maximum diastolic blood pressure (DBP) categories. The matrix cells specify the BP category severity for the SBP and the DBP combination. The category severity defines the MEC referral level.

Table 4-4.　Referral levels for blood pressure (adults)[1]

Systolic	Diastolic				
	<80	80-89	90-99	100-119	>/=120
<120	1	2	3	4	5
120-139	2	2	3	4	5
140-159	3	3	3	4	5
160-209	4	4	4	4	5
>/= 210	5	5	5	5	5

[1] Based on the Seventh Report of the Joint National Committee on the Prevention, Detection, Evaluation, and Treatment of High Blood Pressure. NIH Publication, 2003.

Table 4-5.　Blood pressure referral levels, category, and action guideline (adults)

Referral level	BP Category	Physician guideline referral action
1	5	Indicates major medical findings (BP) that warrant immediate attention by a health care provider.
2	3 & 4	Indicates major medical findings (BP) that warrant attention by a health care provider within the next 2 weeks. These findings are expected to cause adverse effects within this time period and they have previously been undiagnosed, unattended, nonmanifested, or not communicated to the examinee by his/her personal health care provider.
2	2	Indicates prehypertensive blood pressure, minor medical findings that an examinee already knows about, and is under care for, or findings that do not require prompt attention by a medical provider prior to a month.
3	1	Indicates no abnormal BP findings.

Table 4-6. Adults BP referral letter comments

BP Category	BP Referral level	Referral statement
5	1	The participant's blood pressure today is severely high.
4	2	The participant's blood pressure today is very high based on the Seventh Report of the Joint National Committee on the Prevention, Detection, Evaluation, and Treatment of High Blood Pressure. NIH Publication, 2003.
3	2	The participant's blood pressure today is high. Based on the Seventh Report of the Joint National Committee on the Prevention, Detection, Evaluation, and Treatment of High Blood Pressure. NIH Publication, 2003.
2	2	The participant's blood pressure today is above normal and is in the prehypertensive range. Based on the Seventh Report of the Joint National Committee on the Prevention, Detection, Evaluation, and Treatment of High Blood Pressure. NIH Publication, 2003.
1	3	The participant's blood pressure today is within the normal range. Based on the Seventh Report of the Joint National Committee on the Prevention, Detection, Evaluation, and Treatment of High Blood Pressure. NIH Publication, 2003.

Table 4-7. Table of blood pressure Report of Findings comment (adults)

Report of Findings level BP category	Report of Findings message – English	Report of Findings message – Spanish
1	Your blood pressure today **is within the normal range**. Based on the Seventh Report of the Joint National Committee on the Prevention, Detection, Evaluation, and Treatment of High Blood Pressure. NIH Publication, 2003.	Su presión de sangre hoy **está dentro del rango normal**. Basado en el Séptimo Informe del Comité Conjunto Nacional de Prevención, Detección, Evaluación y Tratamiento de la Alta Presión Sanguínea. Publicación del NIH, 2003.
2	Your blood pressure today is **above normal and is in the prehypertensive range**. Based on the Seventh Report of the Joint National Committee on the Prevention, Detection, Evaluation, and Treatment of High Blood Pressure. NIH Publication, 2003.	Su presión de sangre hoy **es por encima de lo normal y está dentro del rango de prehipertensión**. Basado en el Séptimo Informe del Comité Conjunto Nacional de Prevención, Detección, Evaluación y Tratamiento de la Alta Presión Sanguínea. Publicación del NIH, 2003.

Table 4-7.   Table of blood pressure Report of Findings comment (adults) (continued)

Report of Findings level BP category	Report of Findings message – English	Report of Findings message – Spanish
3	Your blood pressure today is **high.** Based on the Seventh Report of the Joint National Committee on the Prevention, Detection, Evaluation, and Treatment of High Blood Pressure. NIH Publication, 2003.	Su presión de sangre hoy es **alta.** Basado en el Séptimo Informe del Comité Conjunto Nacional de Prevención, Detección, Evaluación y Tratamiento de la Alta Presión Sanguínea. Publicación del NIH, 2003.
4	Your blood pressure today is **very high.** Based on the Seventh Report of the Joint National Committee on the Prevention, Detection, Evaluation, and Treatment of High Blood Pressure. NIH Publication, 2003.	Su presión de sangre hoy es **muy alta.** Basado en el Séptimo Informe del Comité Conjunto Nacional de Prevención, Detección, Evaluación y Tratamiento de la Alta Presión Sanguínea. Publicación del NIH, 2003.
5	Your blood pressure today is **severely** high.	Su presión de sangre hoy es **severamente alta.**

(Note: ROF level number 5 should **not** have the NIH Publication referenced.)

4.4.2   Blood Pressure Referrals – Children

Children's normal blood pressures vary by age, weight, and height. Referral comments and Report of Findings comments are shown in Tables 4-8 and 4-9.

The table for children's blood pressures is found in Appendix A, Child Blood Pressure Values.

Table 4-8. Referral comments for blood pressure (children)

BP Category	Referral level	Referral statement*
4	1	The participant's blood pressure is **very high** based on the 1996 update of the Task Force Report on High Blood Pressure in Children and Adolescents.*
3	2	The participant's blood pressure is **high** based on the 1996 update of the Task Force Report on High Blood Pressure in Children and Adolescents.*
2	3	The participant's blood pressure is **normal but at the high end of normal** based on the 1996 update of the Task Force Report on High Blood Pressure in Children and Adolescents.*
1	3	The participant's blood pressure is **normal** based on the 1996 update of the Task Force Report on High Blood Pressure in Children and Adolescents.*

* National High Blood Pressure Education Program Working Group on Hypertension Control in Children and Adolescents. Update on the 1987 Task Force Report on High Blood Pressure in Children and Adolescents: A Working Group Report from the National High Blood Pressure Education Program. *Pediatrics*. 1996; 11:649-658.

Table 4-9. Table of blood pressure Report of Findings comments (children)

Report of Findings level BP Category	Report of findings message
1	Your child's blood pressure today **is within the normal range.***
2	Your child's blood pressure today **is normal but at the high end of normal range.***
3	Your child's blood pressure today is **high.***
4	Your child's blood pressure today is **very high.***

* National High Blood Pressure Education Program Working Group on Hypertension Control in Children and Adolescents. Update on the 1987 Task Force Report on High Blood Pressure in Children and Adolescents: A Working Group Report from the National High Blood Pressure Education Program. *Pediatrics*. 1996; 11:649-658.

4.5   Observation Referrals

Observation referrals are not linked to specific examination data. An observation referral includes any observation by the technician or other examination staff about an SP's condition that may require attention by the physician. An observation referral is sent through the ISIS process from any examination component examiner and may be initiated during the examination, but is sent after the component examination is completed and the SP has left the component room. The examiner initiating the observation enters a message in the observation box and sends it electronically to the physician. The observation sets a flag in the physician component and coordinator applications and SPs are not checked out of the MEC until the physician reviews and acts on this observation. Examples of observations include information from a dietary interviewer when children or adult SPs are thought to be malnourished, or mental health observations from a MEC interviewer. The physician will discuss the issue with the SP and refer as deemed medically necessary.

4.6   Mental Health Observation Referrals

The confidential health and lifestyle interview conducted at the MEC by specially trained interviewers are administered to SPs 12 years and older. The MEC physicians are responsible for determining the need for referrals in two sections of this interview, and include: (1) Depression Screening, and (2) Cognitive Functioning.

The MEC interviewer asks the physician to see any SP who meets criteria for a potential mental health problem. The MEC interviewer protocol directs him or her to inform the physician with regard to the reasons and circumstances that the MEC interviewer may ask the physician to see an SP. In addition to the reasons stated in these instructions, the MEC interviewer may ask the physician to see an SP to evaluate a potential MH issue at other times.

4.6.1   MEC Interviewer Depression Screening

Certain information volunteered or reported during the mental health interview will initiate an automatic electronic mental health observation notification from the MEC interviewer to the MEC physician application. The question asked by the MEC interviewer during the depression screener questionnaire that would prompt an observation to the physician for mental health assessment is the following:

- DPQ090: Over the **last 2 weeks**, how often have you been bothered by the following problem: Thoughts that you would be better off dead or hurting yourself in some way? The response categories for this question are:

    - Not at all;

    - Several days;

    - More than half the days; and

    - Nearly every day.

Responses of several days, more than half the days, and nearly every day require a physician referral for a mental health consultation. If the SP says he or she thought about it only one time in the last 2 weeks, the interviewer codes the response as "several days."

The physician will code the observation as "action required," which will cause ISIS to alert the coordinator that the physician needs to meet with the SP. The physician is responsible for assessing the mental health problem and facilitating a referral, if needed. The Mental Health Referral is a separate referral screen, as shown in Exhibit 4-2, below.

4.6.1.1   Suicidal Ideation

The MEC physician is not responsible for making psychiatric diagnoses; however, thoughts and plans for suicide should be considered seriously. The MEC physician should assess the need for a mental health referral for those who have either reported or voluntarily disclosed recent suicidal ideations or attempts.

Protocol for a MEC physician receiving an observation from the mental health interview:

- Assess if the SP is currently suicidal. Ask the SP if she or he is depressed or thinking about suicide now. If so, then probe as to whether she or he has a plan and/or set a time for doing this. A person who is suicidal with a plan to kill at a definite time is a **psychiatric emergency**, and a Level 1 referral.

Exhibit 4-2. Mental health referral screen

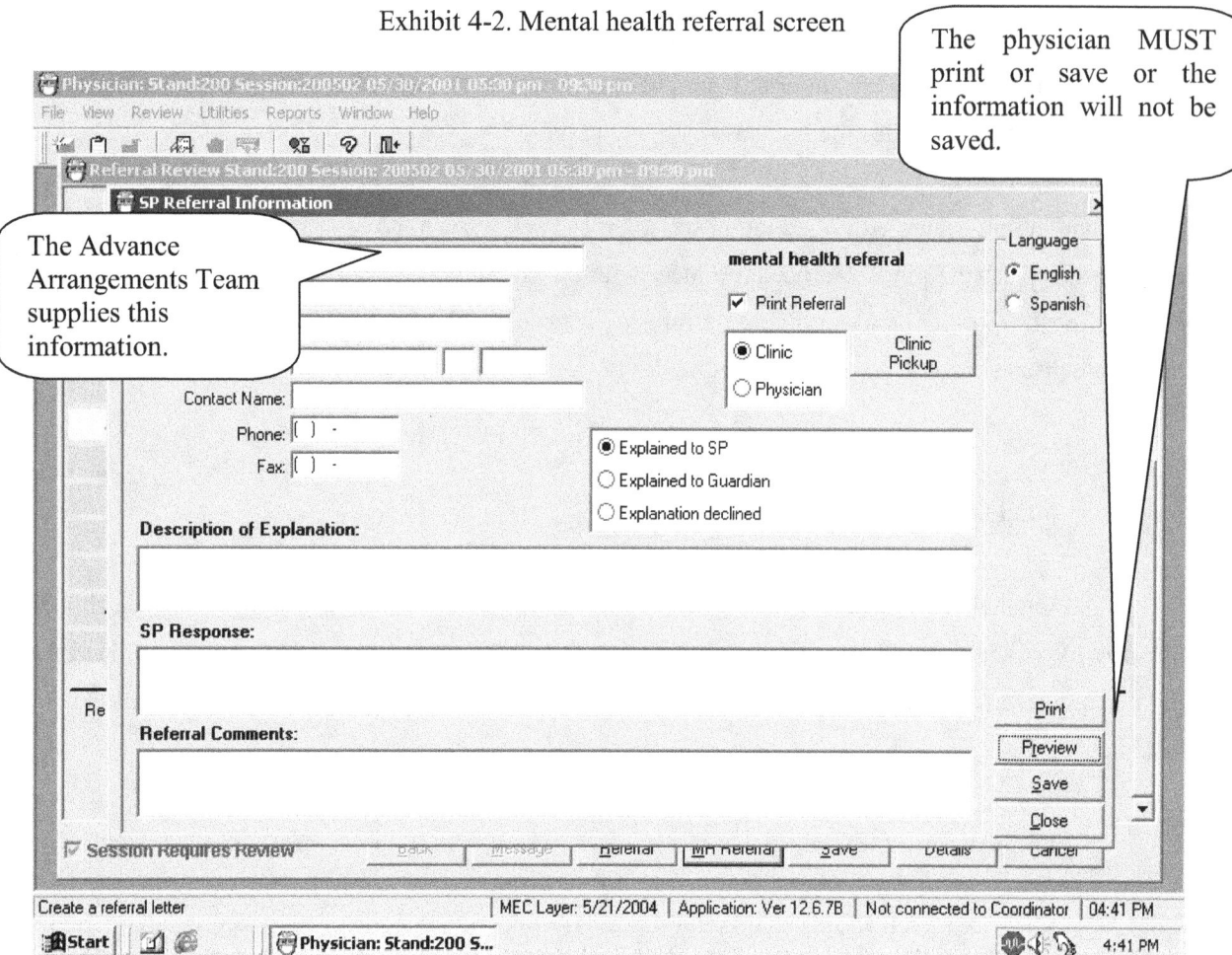

Protocol for a participant who is in imminent danger:

- If the SP is currently under psychiatric care, ask the SP for permission to call the mental health care provider. The physician should negotiate a follow up consultation with the provider. If the participant does not have a provider, call the **referral center provided by the advance arrangements team.**

Protocol for a participant who is not in imminent danger:

- If the SP is under the care of a psychiatrist or other mental health care provider, there may be no need to refer unless the participant provides some indication that his or her symptoms are worsening.

- If the SP has not seen a health professional for suicidal thoughts, then refer him or her to the specific clinics or crisis hotline **provided by the advance arrangements team.**

For minors under 18 years of age, the initial assessment should be done with the youth in private. If a referral is necessary, the participant's parent/guardian must be notified.

4.6.1.2   Homicidal Ideations/Threats

Threats to kill a person or person(s) should be considered seriously. The MEC physician should judge the mental stability of the participant. The physician should ask about the specific plan for carrying out the threat and the timeframe. A homicidal threat with a lethal weapon and plan must be reported to the 911 system.

4.6.1.3   Reporting Child Abuse

If a minor reports that he or she has been abused, the MEC physician should document the nature of the abuse. If warranted, the MEC physician should call **Child Protective Services at the number provided by the NHANES Advance Arrangements Team.** If the physician is unsure whether or not to refer, the physician should discuss the case with a social worker at Child Protective Services. When presenting the case, the MEC physician should not use the child's name or any other identifier. If the social worker and physician agree that the referral to CPS should be made, the physician may provide the name and address of the child.

4.6.2   Cognitive Functioning Referrals

Cognitive measures testing is administered to a subset of the NHANES sample population, adults aged 60 years and older to evaluate executive functioning, memory, and processing speed. Three brief cognitive tests were added to the MEC Interview for these SPs in 2011: (1) the CERAD Word List Learning Test, involving a word list in which recall is assessed after three learning trials and delayed recall; (2) WAIS-III Digit Symbol Substitution Test; and (3) an Animal Fluency test. The MEC interviewer introduces the cognitive tests by conducting a pretest: The SP is asked to name two or more articles of clothing; and the SP is asked to demonstrate the Digit Symbol-Coding test using five symbols. The SP is referred to the physician for a consultation if:

1.   A participant is unable to complete the pretest for verbal fluency, (cannot name two or more articles of clothing) OR:

2.   The participant cannot perform the pretest for the Digit Symbol Substitution Test – (cannot correctly write the symbol for each number in all five sample boxes) OR:

3.   The SP is visibly distressed by any aspect of the cognitive functioning tests.

If any of the above three conditions are met, the MEC interviewer will notify the MEC physician of a need for a consultation with the SP via the observation notification system. The MEC physician will discuss possible memory problems with the participant and determine need for a referral. If the physician deems a referral is necessary, the NHANES medical officer will facilitate referral for the SP. In this case, the physician will insert "Kathryn Porter, MD" and phone number 1-800-452-6115 on the referral letter field. The MEC physician should document the encounter with an SP by either entering information describing the reason no referral was given in the physician Mental Health (MH) Observation box, or by completing an MH referral (Exhibit 4-2, shown earlier).

4.7 Physician Application Referral Procedures

The physician referral process is fully automated and supported by the physician ISIS application and the coordinator application.

The "Sessions Requiring Review" box is displayed every time the physician logs on to the application, and the physician must review these sessions (Exhibit 4-3). When the ISIS application first opens for the physician component, the "Sessions Requiring Review" screen opens by default. The purpose of this screen is to prompt the physician to complete reviews for SPs in all previous sessions. The physician can select which sessions to review.

- When the physician's application is opened, the "Sessions Requiring Review" pick list is displayed. If the physician does not want to review referrals at this time, this screen may be closed by clicking on the "x" in the upper right corner or by clicking "Cancel" in the lower right corner.

- The top part of the screen displays the current stand.

- The lower part of the screen displays the Sessions Review.

- To view all sessions in the current stand, leave the box for "Sessions Requiring Review" unchecked. All sessions in the current stand will be displayed.

- To review a specific session, highlight and double click on that session and that session will be displayed.

- Click "Cancel" to exit without viewing any sessions.

- Close the screen when completed.

Exhibit 4-3. Review all MEC sessions in the current stand

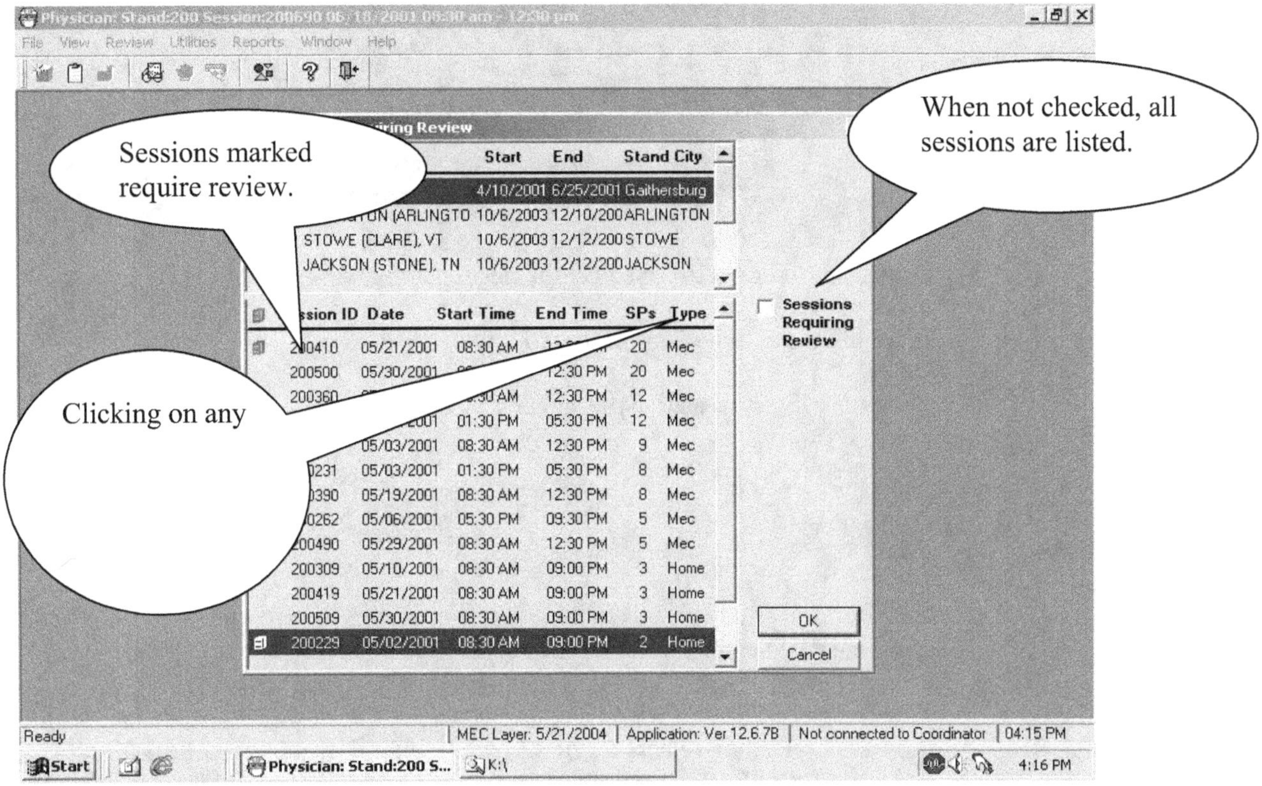

4.7.1 Data Entry Screens for Referrals

The following sections describe the ISIS screens and data entry process related to physician referrals. There are three types of screens related to referral: "Sessions Requiring Review," "Review in Box," and "Referral Review."

4.7.2 Review Menu

The review toolbar selection (Exhibit 4-4) has several review options:, Referral Review, SP History, Review Other Sessions, and Physician Lookup. Each of these options is described in the following sections.

Exhibit 4-4. Review menu for selecting referral review

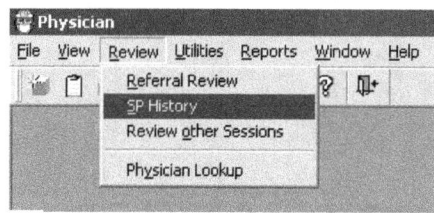

- Use this drop-down list to select the desired activity.

- Highlight the activity by pointing to it with the pointer.

- Click the activity to access the screens.

4.7.3   Review Box

- The Referral Review box option is the screen where all SPs who require an assessment of the need for a referral can be viewed.

- To access the Review Inbox box, first access the desired session (see Exhibit 4-3, shown earlier), then select "Review" (see Exhibit 4-4, shown earlier) from the toolbar, and last, select "Referral Review" from the drop-down list (Exhibit 4-5).

- This will access the referral review requirements for the current session.

Exhibit 4-5. Referral Review selection screen

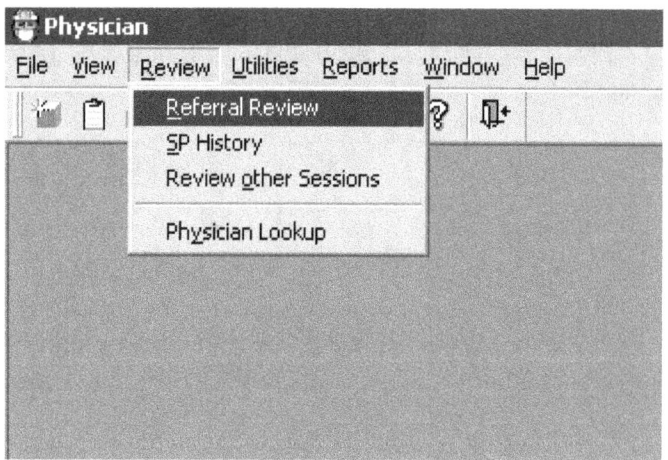

4.7.4   Review Other Sessions

The "Sessions Requiring Review" is accessed from the "Review Other Sessions" drop-down list under the "Review" selection on the toolbar. The "Sessions Requiring Review" screens inform physicians which MEC sessions remain to be reviewed. The purpose of the review is to assure that all referrals are completed. This is especially important since some referrals may not be able to be completed while SPs are still available on the MEC. Physicians mark appropriate boxes about their referral decision for each SP.

Exhibit 4-6 shows the review selection, and drop-down selection list for "Review Other Sessions" option that accesses the Sessions Requiring Review.

Exhibit 4-6. Review other sessions

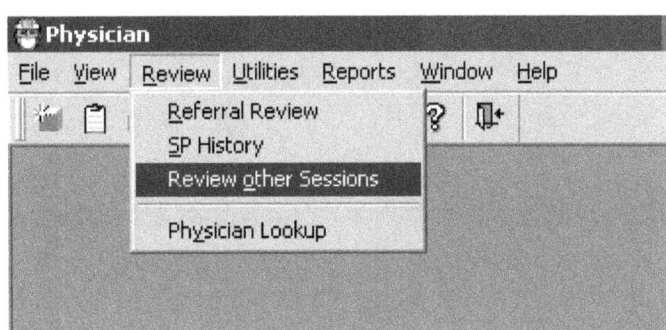

- When the "Review Other Sessions" option is clicked, the "Sessions Requiring Review" screen drop-down list is accessed. From this screen, physicians make choices about which sessions need to be reviewed.

4.7.5   Sessions Requiring Review

The top part of the "Sessions Requiring Review" screen (Exhibit 4-7) displays the current stand location and number. The bottom part of the screen displays various sessions in the stand, depending on how they are selected by the physician.

Exhibit 4-7. MEC Sessions requiring review

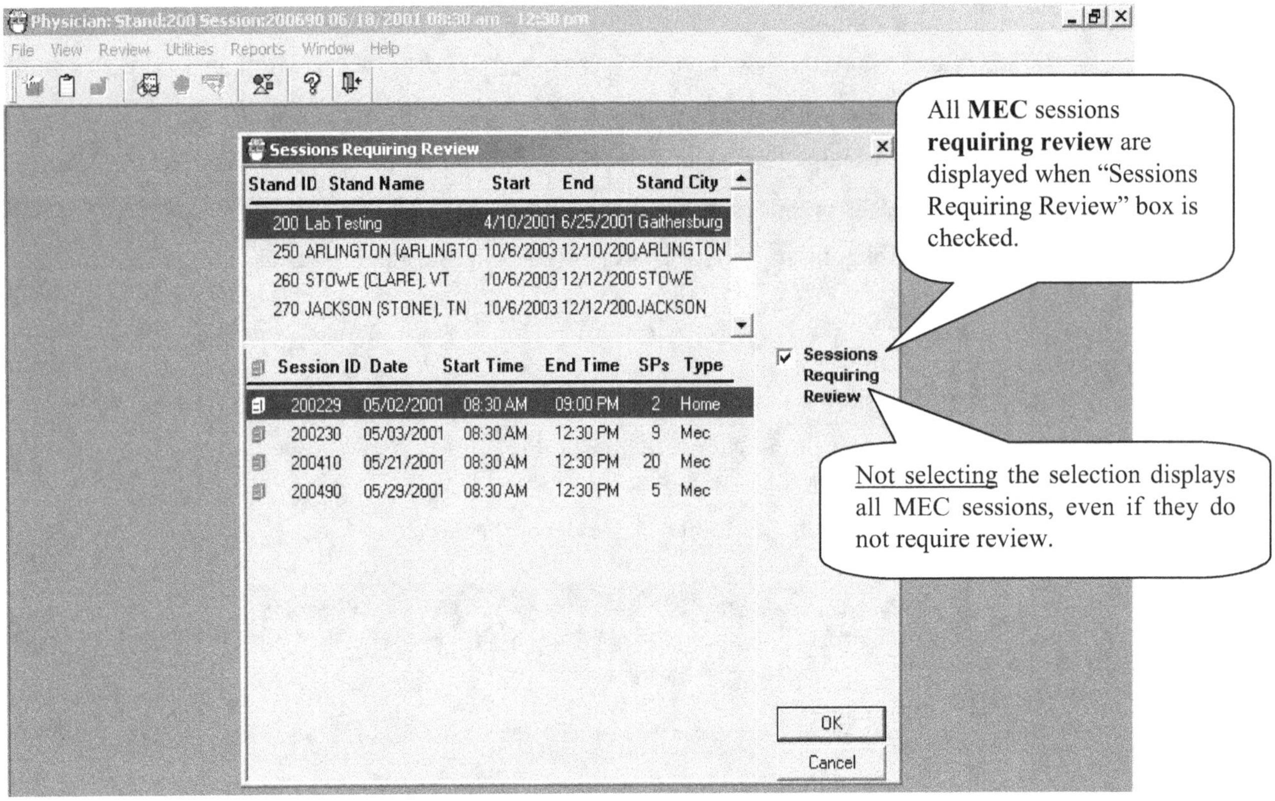

- When the "Sessions Requiring Review" box is checked, all MEC sessions that require review are displayed.

- Referrals posted in the "Review Box" that the physician has not reviewed causes the application screen to display a **red marking beside the session indicating that the session requires review (Exhibit 4-8).**

- The **red mark remains** beside this session until the physician reviews all referrals in the session.

- When all referrals are completed or reviewed, the system removes the red flag.

4.7.6   Referral Review Inbox Screen

- The "Referral Review" box (Exhibit 4-8) has the stand and session numbers on the top bar.

- Names of SPs requiring review are highlighted in red. The boxes for components requiring review are enabled. All other boxes are disabled or "grayed out."

- Note also that the SPs name is in red when a review is required.

Exhibit 4-8. SPs referred back to MD for review for referral determination

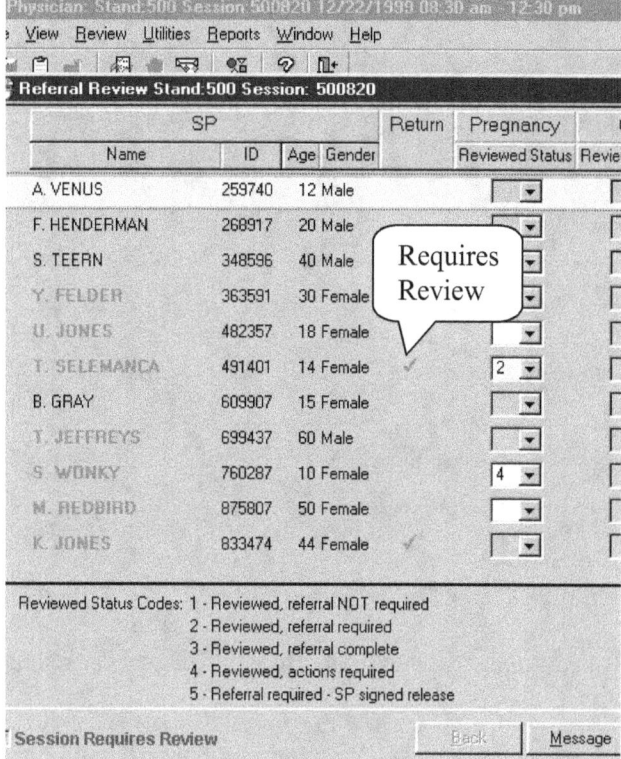

4.7.7 Selecting SP for Detailed Referral Review

To complete the referral, the physician selects each SP in turn who has an indication that a review for referral determination is needed. The selection is made from the Referral Review screen (Exhibit 4-9).

Exhibit 4-9. SP Selection from review in box

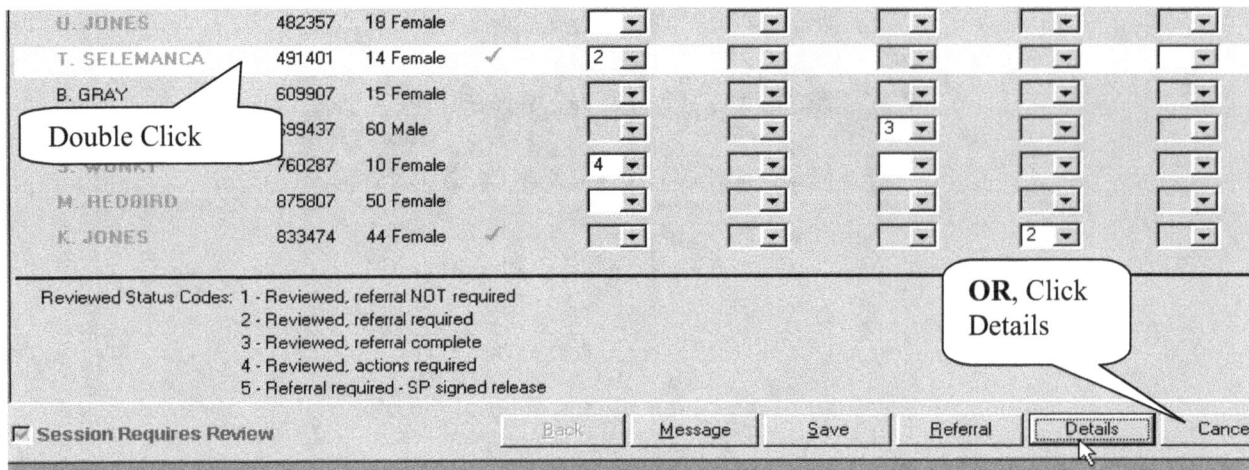

- To select the SP for review, move the cursor over the desired name.

- Highlight the name of the SP to be reviewed.

- Double click on the SP name, or, click the "Details" radio button.

- If you want to close a session before saving the results, a message will be displayed: "Do you want to save changes?" See Exhibit 4-10.

- Click "Yes" to save and close this box. If all status codes are 1 and 3, the "Session Requires Review" box will be unchecked and the red flag will be removed from the session requiring review list. See Exhibit 4-11.

Exhibit 4-10. Warning to save changes

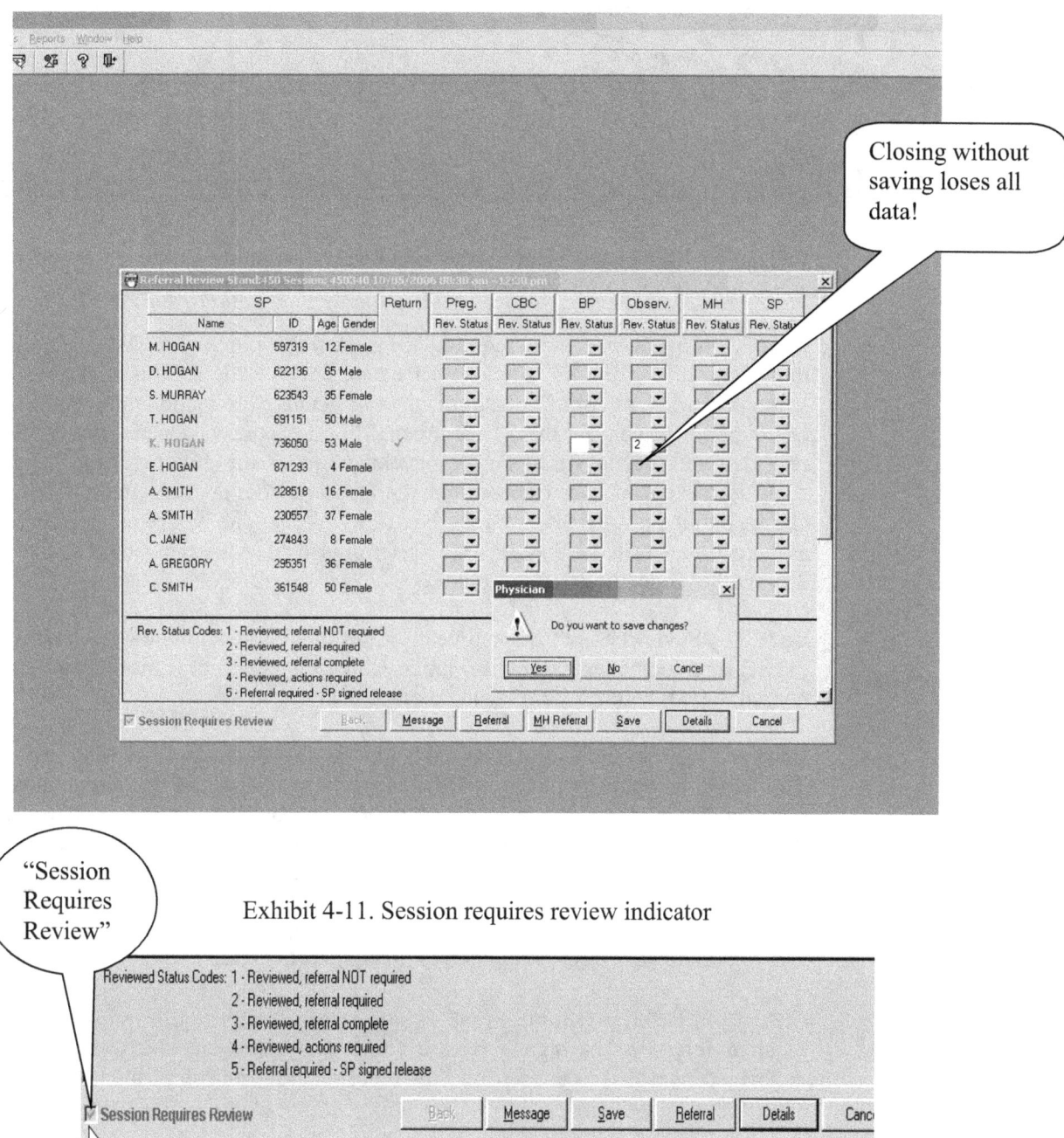

Exhibit 4-11. Session requires review indicator

- A box at the bottom left of the screen is checked if the session requires review. The box is unchecked if no review is required.

- This box is especially useful if there is a long list of SPs. If the box is not checked, there is no need to scroll through the SP list.

- The "Reviewed Status Codes" are listed at the bottom left of the screen (Exhibit 4-12).

Exhibit 4-12. Reviewed status codes legend

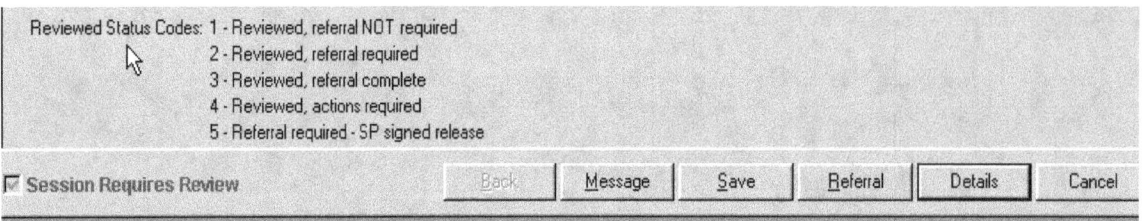

- Code 1 – "Reviewed, referral not required": If findings were reviewed but the situation does not require a referral, select Code 1 from the drop-down menu.

- Code 2 – "Reviewed, referral required": If a referral is required but there is not enough time to do it or if the SP is in another exam, check Code 2. This keeps the referral session active. A referral Code 2 turns the physicians examination progress box on the coordinator's screen (for that SP) to green. This alerts the coordinator that the SP must return to see the physician before checking out of the MEC. (If the SP has not completed the physicians exam component, the box does not turn green. When the SP checks into the physicians exam the box turns green). The box remains green as long as there are referrals for that SP with a referral Code 2. After the code is changed from 2 to another code, the box turns blue.

- Code 3 – "Reviewed, referral complete": After the physician reviews the referral, sees the SP, and completes the referral letter, Code 3 is checked. If no other referrals are needed, the session will be considered complete.

- Code 4 – "Reviewed, action required": This is similar but not the same as Code 2. This code is marked when the SP has been reviewed and a referral generated; however, the physician wants to take further action but has not been able to complete the action at this time. This situation could occur when the physician needs to telephone a health care provider but has been unable to complete the process. This may be carried over to the next day, or the next session. When Code 4 is checked, the SP may be checked out of the MEC but this session continues to be flagged, requiring review until this and other referrals are coded as 1 or 3.

- Code 5 – "Referral required – SP signed release": When SPs refuse to accept a required referral, they sign a release form. The physician checks Code 5 which removes the red flag on the session if all other referrals are complete.

4.7.8   ISIS Message

To assure that SPs see the physician prior to leaving the MEC, the physician can send a message to the coordinator to specify a time to send the SP to the physician examination room to complete the referral (Exhibit 4-13).

Exhibit 4-13. Message to coordinator

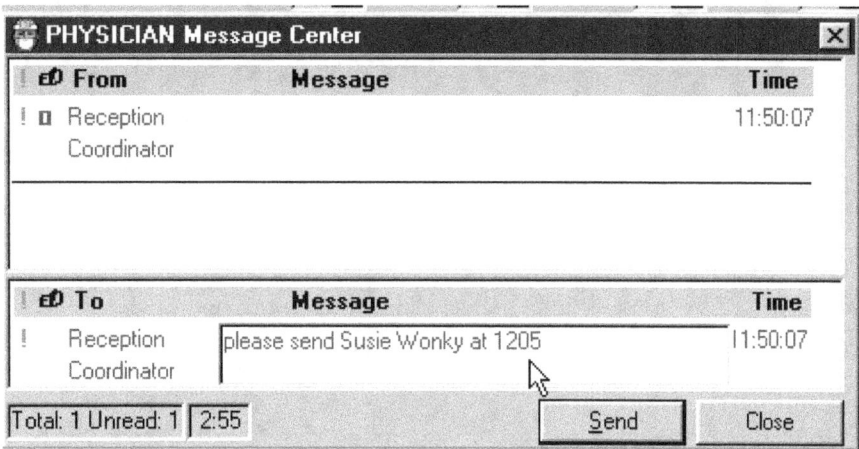

- Notify the coordinator when it is a good time to complete this referral.

- Click "Message" from the tool bar utilities, type a message, and send to the coordinator.

4.7.9   **NHANES Release Form for SPs Refusing Referrals**

- SPs who decline or refuse a medical referral, are asked to sign the NHANES Release Form (Exhibit 4-14). The date and stand number must be completed. The form is available in English and Spanish.

- This form is available for printing in the "Forms" directory.

- Ask the SP to place a checkmark next to the correct ending for the reference sentence:

  - "This is to certify that against the advice of the staff doctor, I."

  - ☐   am leaving the Mobile Exam Center

  - ☐   am removing (name of sample person)

  - ☐   choose no further medical referral or immediate followup.

- Ask the SP to sign this form.

- Obtain a witness signature for the form.

Exhibit 4-14. NHANES release form

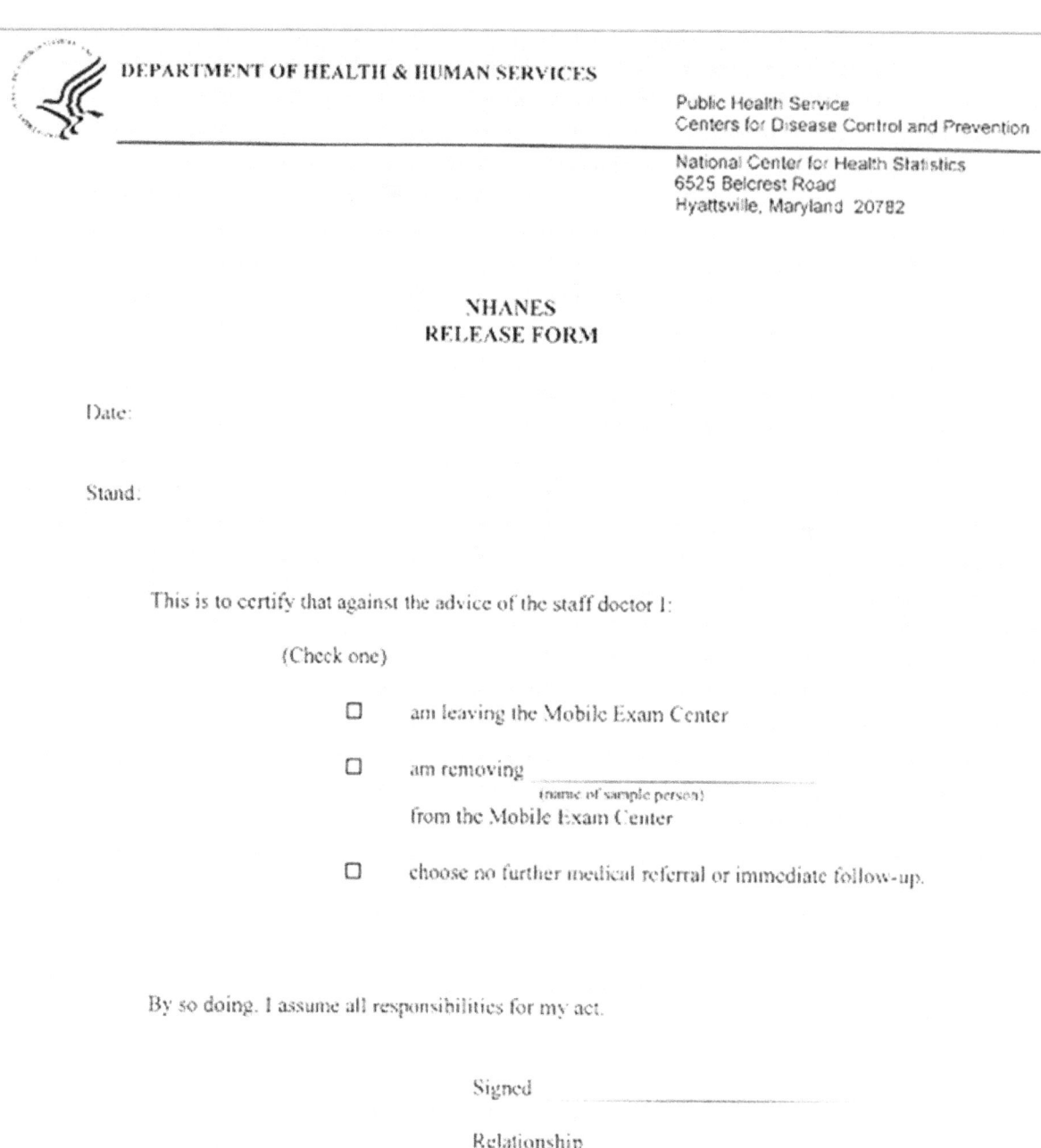

DEPARTMENT OF HEALTH & HUMAN SERVICES

Public Health Service
Centers for Disease Control and Prevention

National Center for Health Statistics
6525 Belcrest Road
Hyattsville, Maryland 20782

**NHANES
RELEASE FORM**

Date:

Stand:

This is to certify that against the advice of the staff doctor I:

(Check one)

☐   am leaving the Mobile Exam Center

☐   am removing _____
                 (name of sample person)
from the Mobile Exam Center

☐   choose no further medical referral or immediate follow-up.

By so doing, I assume all responsibilities for my act.

Signed _____

Relationship _____

Witness _____

4.7.10   Review in Box for Pregnancy Details

The potential data for referral are selected from tabs for each SP that is referred: Pregnancy, CBC, BP, LED, and Observations (Exhibit 4-15).

Exhibit 4-15. Details for pregnancy referral

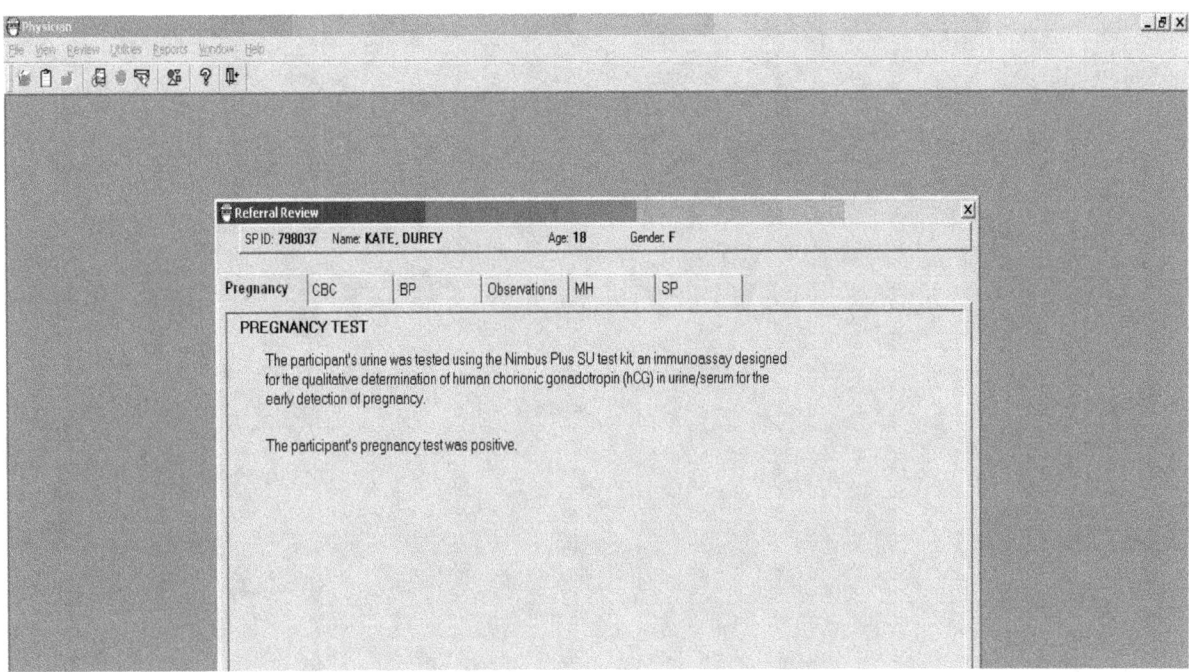

- If the "Pregnancy" tab is checked, the results of the pregnancy test in the lab are displayed. The results can only be one of the following for pregnancy:

    - The pregnancy test is negative;

    - The pregnancy test is positive; or

    - The pregnancy test is invalid.

- Complete the referral as appropriate (Exhibit 4-16).

4.7.11   Review in Box for CBC Details

Exhibit 4-16. Details of complete blood count referral (1)

Referral Review						X
SP ID: **481844** Name: **R2, SD**			Age: **29**	Gender: **F**		

Pregnancy   CBC |BP | Observations | MH | SP |

CBC

Complete Blood Count	Result	Units	Flag	Reference Range
White Blood Count	5.1	(x10^9/L)		4.1 - 12.9
Lymphocytes	31.3	(%)		14.1 - 47.6
Monocytes	0	(%)	Low	3.8 - 11.6
Neutrophils	49.1	(%)		39.8 - 78.1
Eosinophils	7.5	(%)	High	0.6 - 7.3
Basophils	1.5	(%)		0.1 - 1.7
Red Blood Count	4.9	(x10^{12}/L)		3.6 - 5.2
NRBC	0.9	(x10^{12}/L)		0 - 0.3
Hemoglobin	13.0	(g/dL)		10.6 - 15.6
Hematocrit	39.8	(%)		32 - 45.9
MCV	81.0	(fL)		74.6 - 98.2
MCH	26.5	(pg)		24.3 - 33.8
MCHC	32.6	(g/dL)		32.1 - 35.3
RDW	21.5	(%)	High	11.4 - 16.3
Platelets	261.0	(x10^9/L)		168 - 441

Suspect Messages

Giant platelets may be present.

This finding was not confirmed by microscopy and follow-up may be necessary.

Close

- Click on the CBC tab to review the results of the MEC laboratory CBC.

- The names of the tests are displayed in the left columns along with the units of measurement.

- The reference ranges are displayed in the far right column.

- The results and units of measurement are displayed in the next two columns.

- The flagged items are displayed as "low, high, and extremely high."

- Complete the referral as necessary.

- The CBC tab will be split into an upper and lower section. The upper section will display the information currently sent to this section. The lower section of the page will display the information below. Both sections should have a scrolling capability and should there be a large amount of information on either section of the page.

- In order to make the physician aware of the CBC results from the new Coulter, we are sending the suspect flags to both the physician component and the ROF. The physician will access these results as they would any CDC results through the "referral review" details for an individual SP in the current session. However, the physician's component should display only the ROF suspect flag explanation, not the suspect flag codes: machine-produced "suspect" messages – i.e., sickled cells, left shift, or giant platelets.

- The displayed suspect messages will appear so that the physician can also see what the SP will receive. The bottom of the page, when any CBC suspect flag explanations are present, should also display the bolded statement **"This finding was not confirmed by microscopy and followup may be necessary."**

4.7.12   Review in Box – Blood Pressure Details

- Click on the blood pressure tab to view the BP results (Exhibit 4-17).

- Complete the referral if necessary and enter the appropriate code.

- The blood pressure in the above example is very high for the age group and is a Level 2 referral. These results are discussed with the SP and the physician gives a Level 2 referral letter to the SP. The SP may take this letter to his or her health care provider.

- Click on the "Close" button to exit from this screen.

Exhibit 4-17. Details of very high blood pressure referral

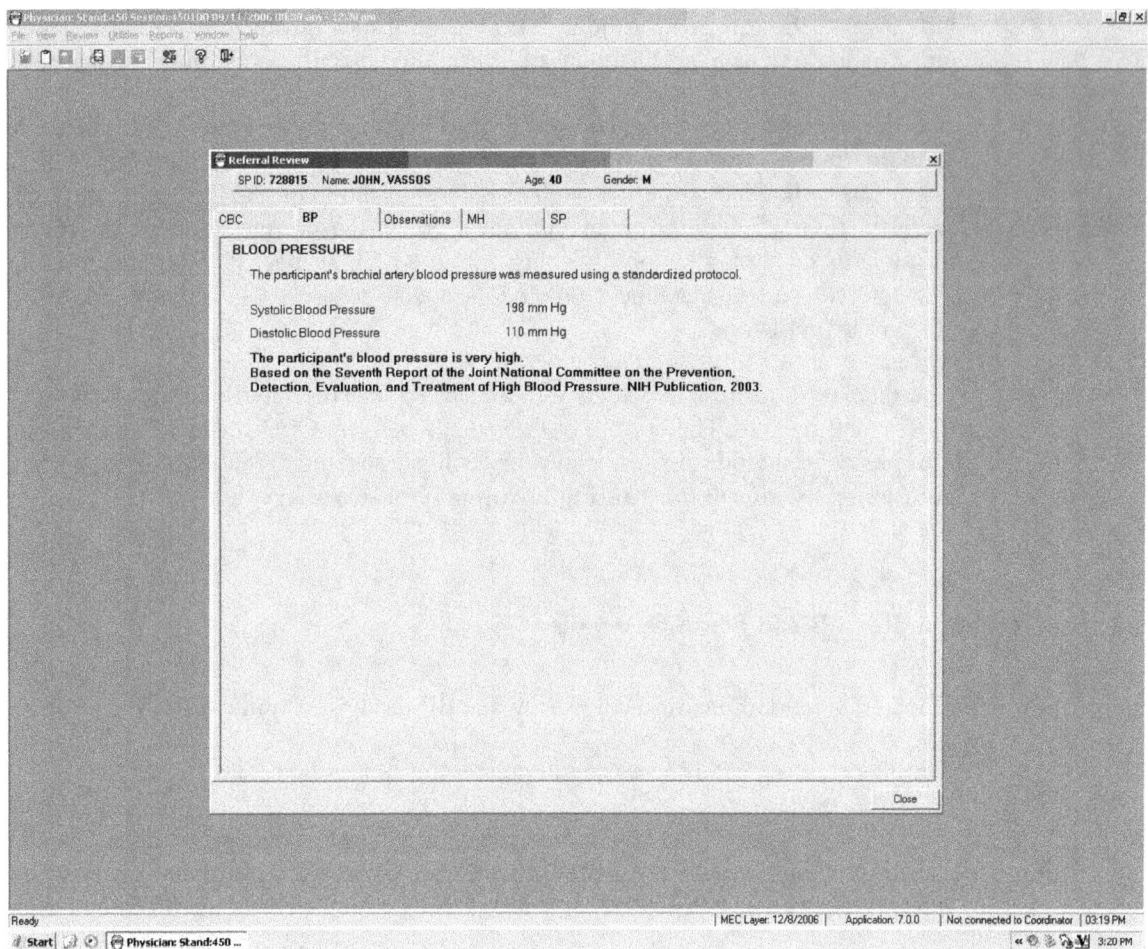

- The blood pressure in Exhibit 4-18 is severely high. This is a Level 1 referral. The physician should try to get an immediate referral to the SP's health care provider or to a local clinic.

- Complete the referral as necessary.

- Click on the "Close" button to exit this screen.

Exhibit 4-18. Details of severely high blood pressure referral

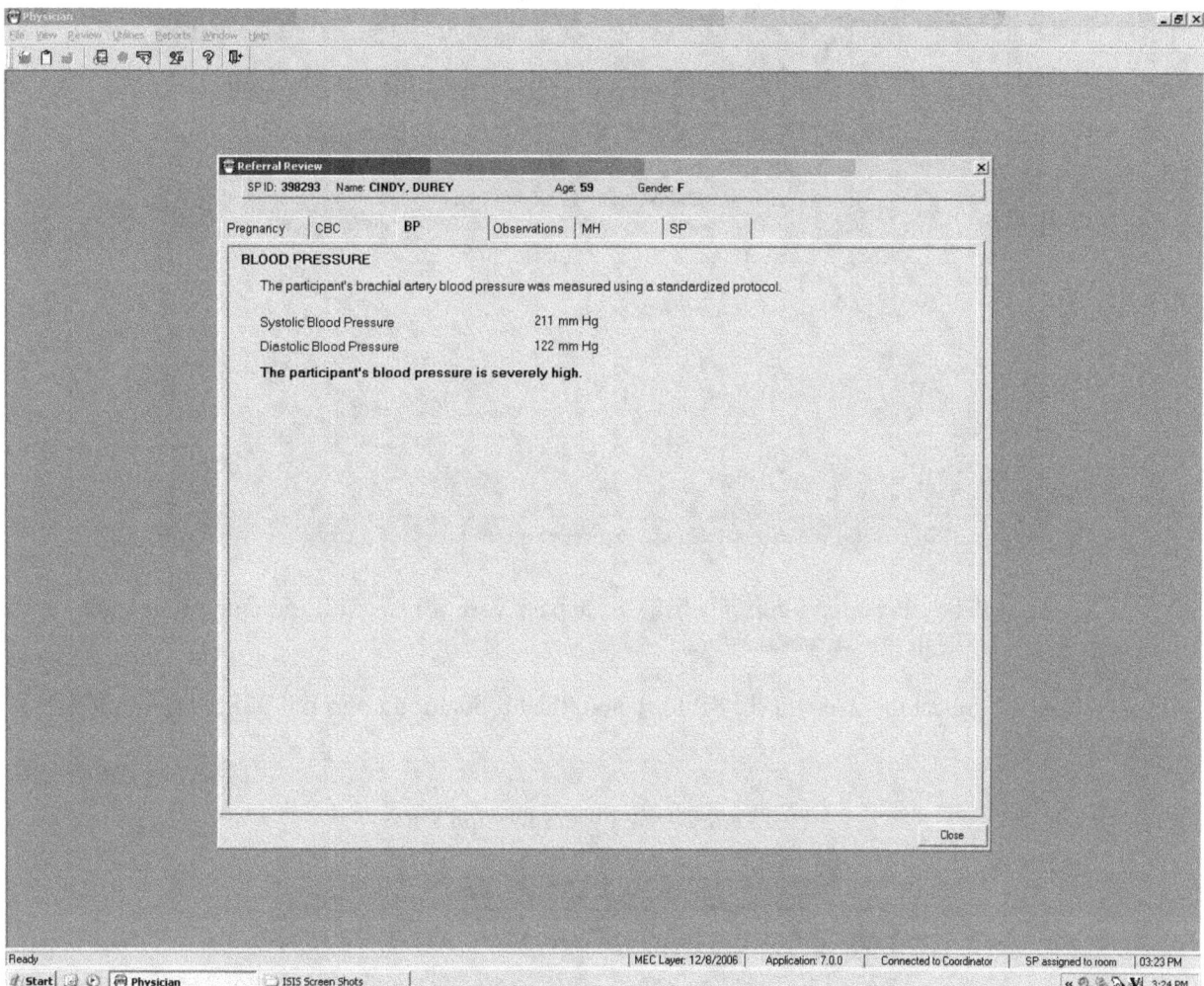

4.8 Observation Referrals

Observation referrals can be displayed by selecting "Observations" from the Utilities toolbar menu. This allows the physician to select any SP from the list of SPs referred for observation. The physician can also select the "Observations" tab from the Review in Box screen for the specific SP being reviewed.

- Select the "Utilities" menu from the toolbar to access the Observations Referral window and then select Observations from the menu (Exhibit 4-19).

Exhibit 4-19. Utilities menu for selecting observations referrals

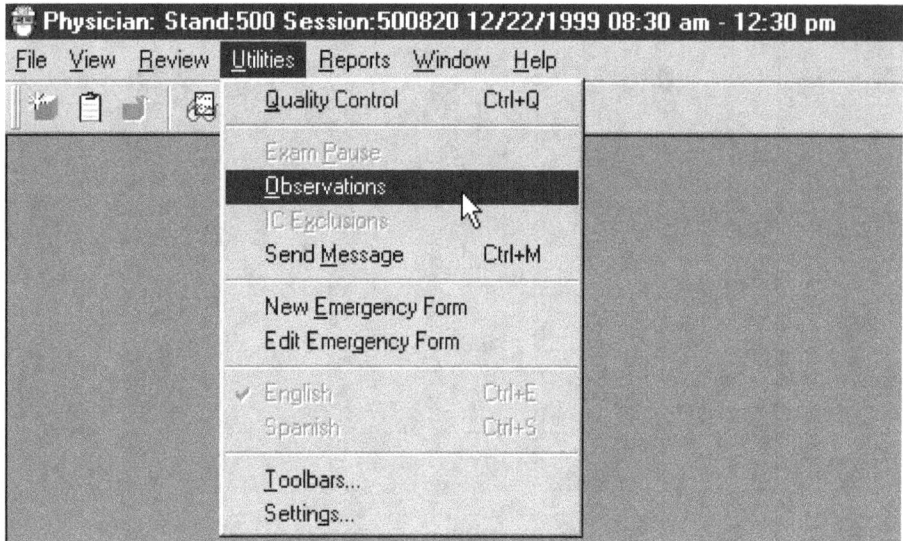

- The SP Observation picklist will appear with a list of all the names and ages of the SPs in the current session.

- Select the name of the SP for whom the observation referral is needed (Exhibit 4-20).

Exhibit 4-20. SP observation picklist

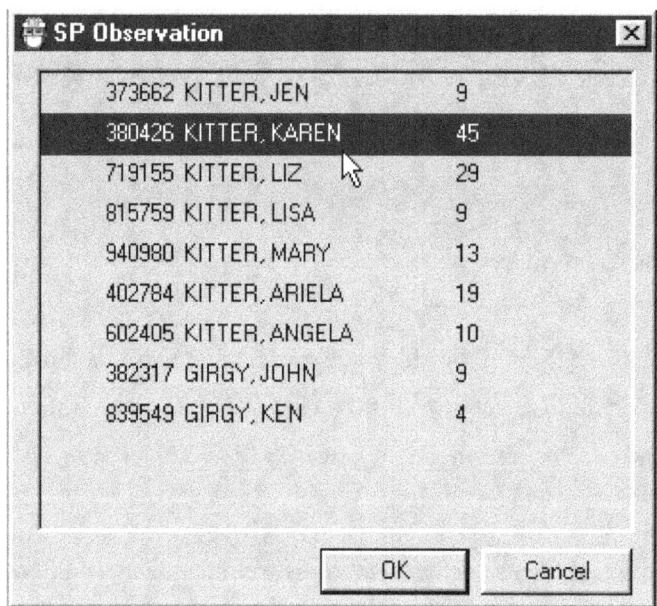

- This is the Observations referral box (Exhibit 4-21) that will be displayed in the other components. The technician will open this box, write the information in the referral information box, and send it to the physician.

- This will be flagged in the physicians exam system and the SP will not be able to leave the MEC until the physician has reviewed this referral.

Exhibit 4-21. Observations referral box

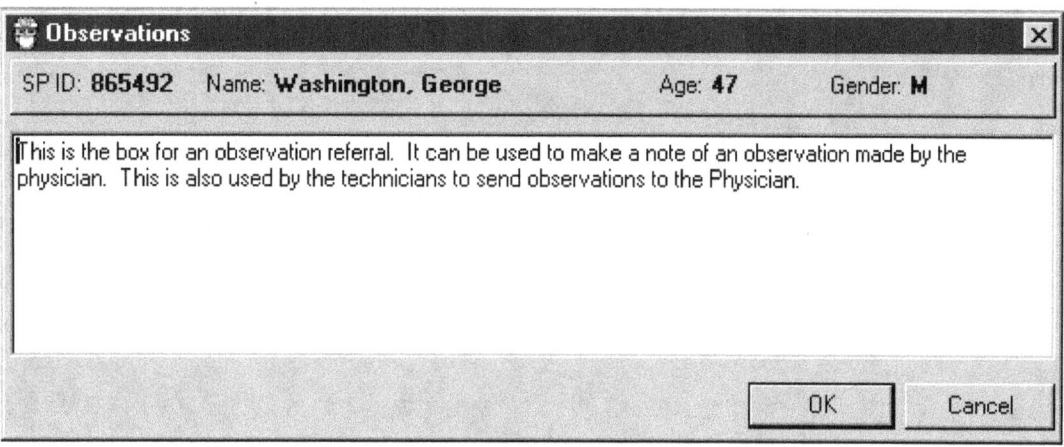

4.8.1 Referral Letter

- When the "Medical Referral" button is clicked, Exhibit 4-22 is displayed. Click on "Clinic Pickup" to view a list of local clinics. Click on "Physician" to see a list of local providers.

- The address and phone number will appear in the appropriate boxes.

- Enter a description of your explanation of the referral to the SP, and how the SP responds.

- The box at the bottom of the screen (Referral Comments) is for entering physician comments. These comments will appear on the second page of the referral letter.

Exhibit 4-22. Clinic pick-up medical referral screen

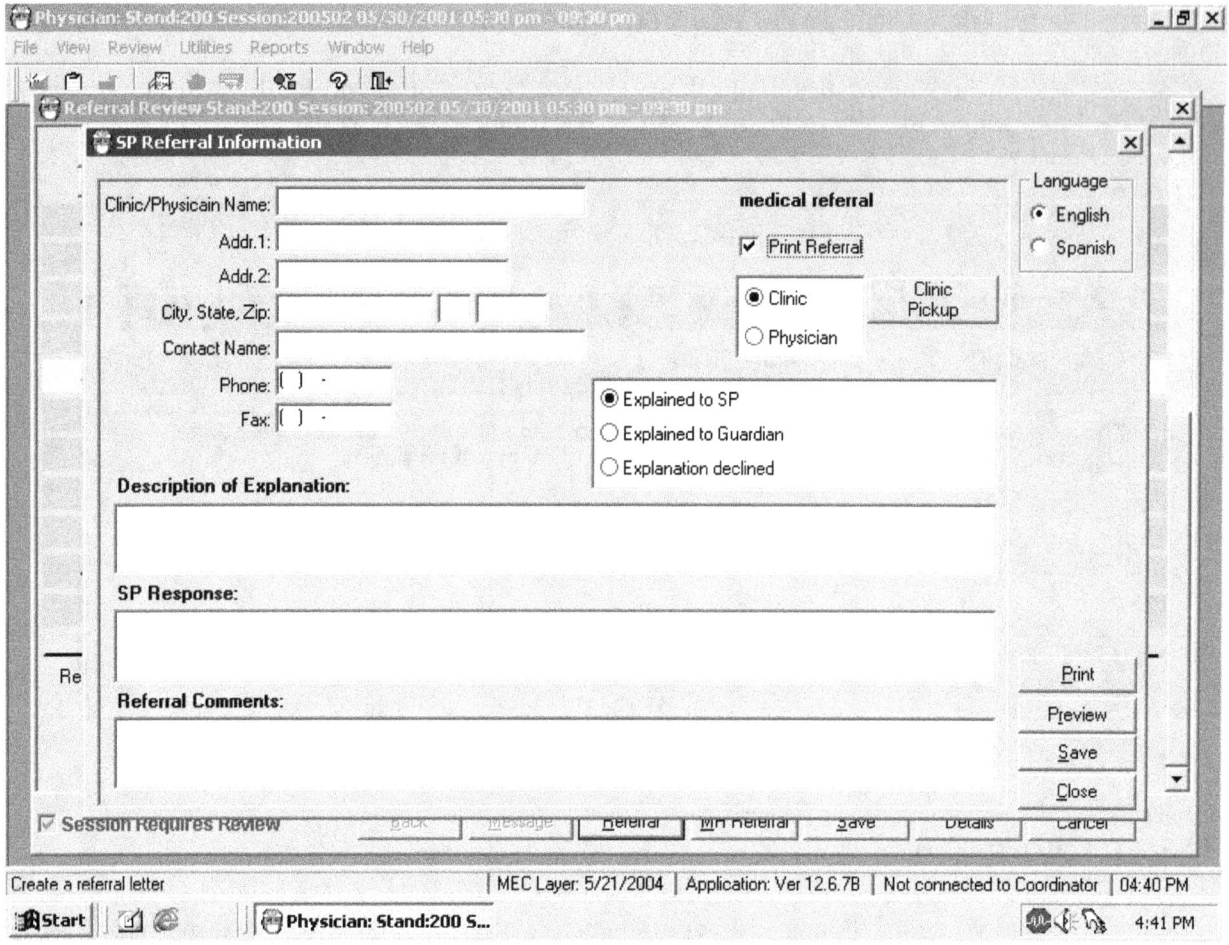

4.8.2   Local Physician Pickup

■   Select the name of the clinic or health care provider (Exhibit 4-23).

Exhibit 4-23. Local physician and clinic pickup referral letter addresses

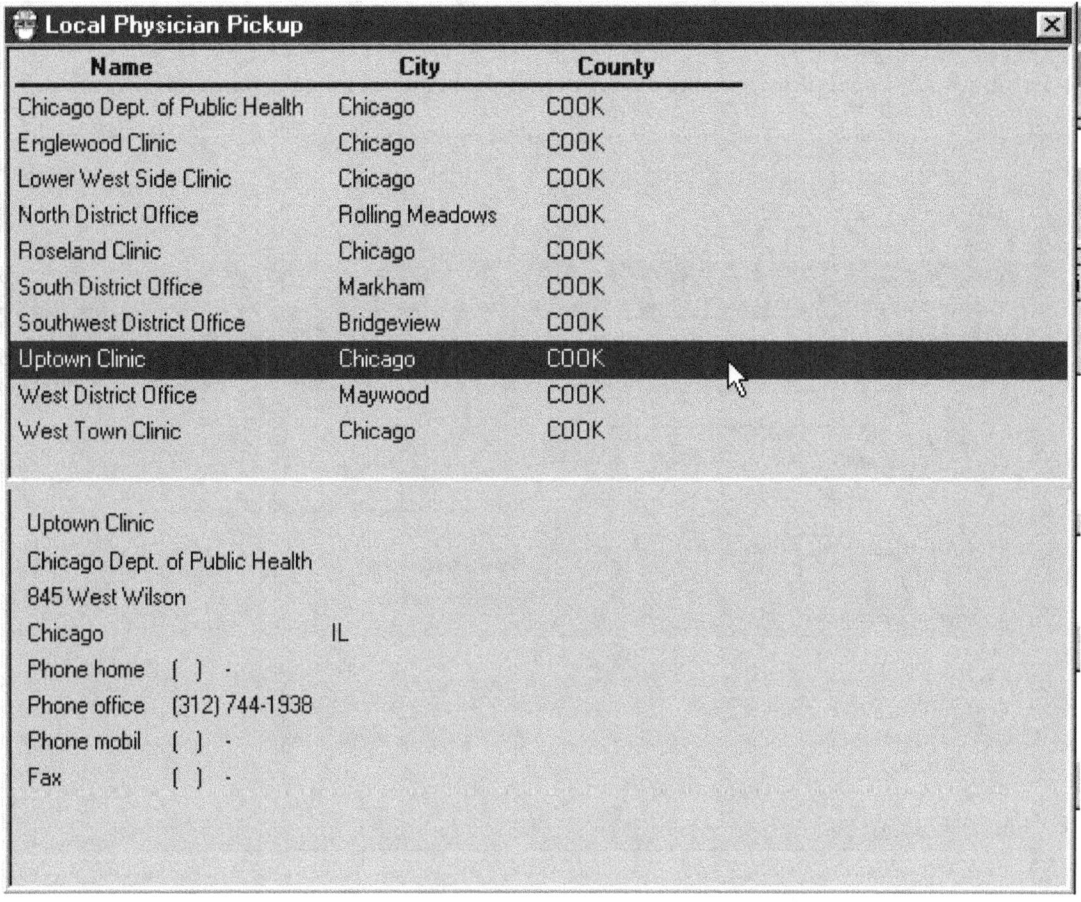

4.8.3 Referral Address Information

- Describe the explanation given to the SP and the SP's response in the appropriate fields. These entries will not appear on the referral letter.

- The "Referral Comments" field may be used to enter comments to the referral physician (Exhibit 4-24).

Exhibit 4-24. Local physician and clinic pickup data entered for referral letter information

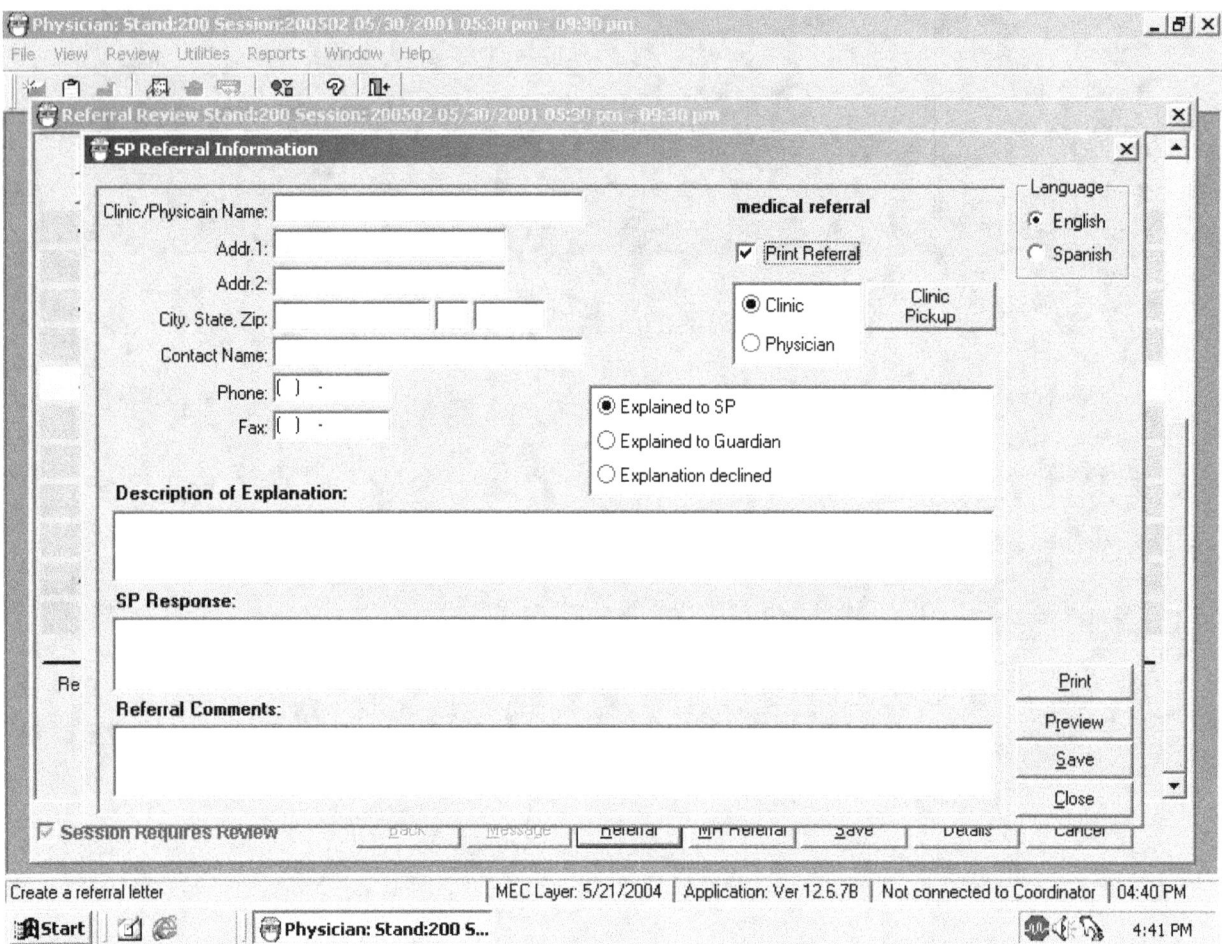

4.8.4 Referral Letter Review

- Select "Preview" from the Session Review in Box screen.

- A preview of the referral letter will be displayed (Exhibit 4-25). Use the scroll bar to view all areas of the letter.

Exhibit 4-25. Preview referral letter

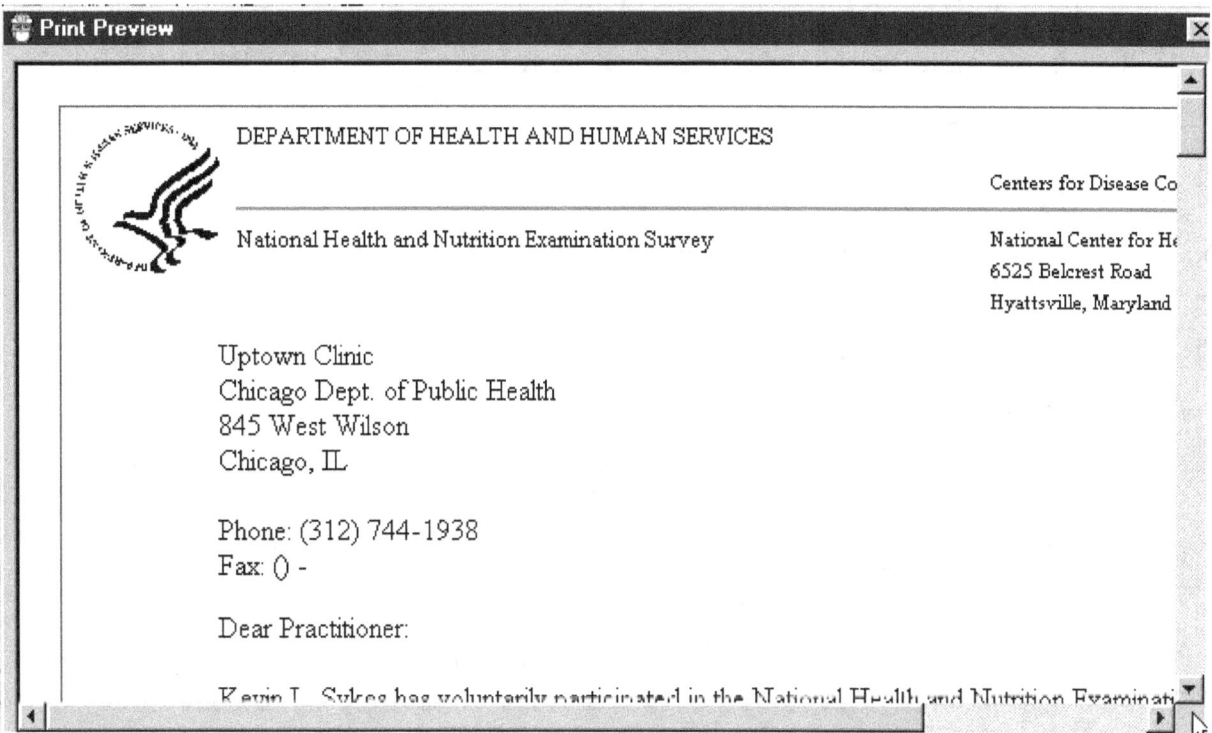

4.8.5   Referral Letter

- The data display for this referral letter (Exhibit 4-26) includes all areas for referral in a single letter.

Exhibit 4-26. Referral letter mock-up

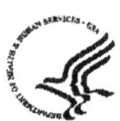 **DEPARTMENT OF HEALTH & HUMAN SERVICES**

Public Health Service
Centers for Disease Control and Prevention

National Center for Health Statistics
6525 Belcrest Road
Hyattsville, Maryland 20782

<Insert Clinics Name> or <SPs Physician>
<Insert Clinic Address>
<Insert Clinic City, ST, Zip>
<Insert Point of Contact>
<Insert Phone Number>

Dear Doctor:

<SP Name> has voluntarily participated in the fourth National Health and Nutrition Examination Survey conducted at special facilities of the U.S. Public Health Service. The objectives of the survey are to obtain information on the health and nutrition status of the U.S. population. As a result of the testing that was done, it was noted that on **<Exam Date>**, a finding was revealed that was outside the survey's medically acceptable range. This finding is described on the attached Referral Comments page.

<Insert the following paragraph for SPs with Blood Pressure Level 1>
As indicated on the Referral Comments page the participant's blood pressure measurements were severely high. The measurements were taken three times; and the values indicated are the average of the last two measures. All survey participants with severely high blood pressure are instructed to see their doctor or clinic the same day, or go to a hospital emergency room to have their blood pressure rechecked.

This examination is intended to collect health measures for research. It is not a complete physical exam. No attempt has been made to diagnose or treat medical conditions of the participants. The findings disclosed to you are done so with the participant's permission.

Should you have any questions, you may contact me at the Mobile Exam Center. The phone number is **<MEC Physician Phone>** until **<MEC Stand End Date>**. After that date you may contact Dr. Kathryn Porter at the National Center for Health Statistics, Monday through Friday 9 AM to 6PM, EST. The toll free number is 1-800-452-6115.

Cordially,

<MEC Physician Name>, M.D.

5. SAFETY ISSUES AND EMERGENCY PROCEDURES

5.1   Safety in the Mobile Examination Center (MEC)

The best approach to emergency situations in the MEC is to prevent problems from developing into emergencies whenever possible, and to be well prepared for those emergencies that cannot be avoided. It is the responsibility of all examination staff members to participate in maintaining safety in the MEC by staying alert for potentially unsafe conditions or unusual sample person (SP) behavior, and by being thoroughly familiar with the current NHANES procedures for emergencies.

Promotion of safety and prevention of accidents and emergencies in the MEC is of particular concern in NHANES in view of the proportion of elderly sample persons that will be participating in the survey. The number of elderly respondents will be significant as a result of an intentional oversampling and removal of the upper age limit on the examination.

5.1.1   Elderly Sample Persons

Care should be taken with all elderly sample persons to minimize confusion and ensure the safe completion of the examination. Elderly SPs should be escorted when moving between exam procedures and the coordinator's area, and should not be left alone for more than a few minutes, such as when changing clothes.

Instructions to elderly SPs should be provided in a clear, calm manner, and repeated as needed. It should not be assumed that the directions are understood until the SP offers an appropriate response. It may be necessary to guide SPs through each step required, such as providing a urine specimen or changing into a gown, to successfully complete a task. If the SP has difficulty understanding or performing tasks, try to offer one instruction or direction at a time and wait until the SP understands before proceeding.

Exam staff should be particularly alert to complaints or concerns from elderly SPs, as they may not clearly communicate the extent of their discomfort or concern. Staff members will need to further investigate SP complaints and refer all potential problems to the MEC physician.

5.1.2   Sample Persons in Wheelchairs

Some SPs may arrive for the examination in wheelchairs, and the exam staff will have to facilitate the SPs' entry into the MEC and their progress through the examination. The field office will alert the MEC manager and coordinator that an examinee uses a wheelchair for mobility so that the handicap lift in trailer 1 can be prepared.

SPs in wheelchairs will enter the MEC through the handicapped access hydraulic lift in trailer 1, and then will be taken to the reception area where the coordinator will check them in and initiate the exam. The MEC trailers are large enough to allow passage of most wheelchairs. If an SP's wheelchair cannot move easily through the MEC, the SP may be transferred to the MEC wheelchair located in the wheelchair-accessible bathroom. If the SP can bear sufficient weight on at least one leg, or can otherwise support him or herself during the transfer, the physician and another exam staff member should assist him or her into the MEC wheelchair to facilitate movement throughout the MEC.

Sample persons who cannot bear most of their weight on one leg and need assistance in transferring to the MEC chair should not be lifted or moved out of their wheelchairs. Lifting or moving SPs without their assistance could result in injury to an SP or staff member and is unwarranted. SPs should remain in their wheelchairs and receive the exams that can be conducted in that position. When the transfer of an SP raises questions, the physician should make the decision to transfer or not transfer an SP.

5.1.3   Children in the MEC

Children in the MEC should be monitored at all times when not participating in an exam component. Young children should not be permitted to walk through the MEC unescorted and should not interfere with the performance of any examinations.

When waiting for an exam, young or unruly children should remain in the reception area under the supervision of the MEC coordinator and assistant coordinator. Other staff members, when available, may be asked to assist the MEC coordinator and assistant coordinator during particularly busy sessions. A limited collection of small toys is available to entertain young children.

Staff members should be alert to the presence of children in the MEC and always investigate the behavior of young children walking unattended through the exam center.

5.2 Safety Precautions

A number of precautions have been taken to promote safety in the exam center.

5.2.1 Mobile Exam Center Preparation

- Fire extinguishers have been placed throughout the MEC to allow rapid response to fire. Exit doors are present in every trailer.

- A drug kit, an automated external defibrillator, two portable oxygen tanks, and portable blood pressure equipment are kept in one box in the physician's exam room in each caravan. All staff must be able to recognize and locate this equipment without delay.

- Pocket masks for CPR are in the following areas: the coordinator's station, vision room, respiratory health room, body measures room, physician's exam room, MEC interview room #2, dietary interview room #1, the staff room, phlebotomy room, body composition room, dental exam room, and the audiometry room.

- The phone number "911" is to be used to activate EMS if applicable for the MEC location. The telephone number and address of the local fire and rescue squad will also be posted at the coordinator's station and in the staff room by the telephone.

- The address of the MEC will be posted in the coordinator's station and staff room so that the location can be reported correctly to EMS.

- The MEC is a "NO SMOKING" facility. Neither staff nor SPs may smoke in the exam center. Should a staff member or SP have the need to smoke, she or he should step outside the MEC.

5.2.2 Mobile Examination Staff Preparation

- All examination staff members are certified in cardiopulmonary resuscitation, Course Level C, and recertified biannually.

- A physician is required to be present when SPs are in the MEC.

- All examination staff are required to be in the MEC while a session is in progress and whenever SPs are in the MEC.

- All staff are required to be thoroughly familiar with the safety issues and emergency procedures.

- Mock emergency drills will be held periodically in the mobile exam center to simulate a medical emergency and permit practice of emergency procedures.

5.2.3   On-Site Preparations at Each Stand

- The field office or the advance arrangements team will contact and meet with local fire and rescue representatives to orient them to the location and structure of the MEC.

- The field office will provide advance notice to the MEC coordinator of any SPs who will require assistance entering or moving through the exam center. The coordinator will inform the MEC manager so that appropriate preparations can be made.

- The physician will review the medication history from the household interview for each SP prior to the examination session in which the SP's appointment is scheduled. The SP medication information can be accessed by the physician in the ISIS Physician's Exam application.

5.3   Reporting SP Problems to the MEC Physician

SPs who report feeling ill or who appear to feel ill should be reported to the MEC physician at the earliest opportunity. At times SPs may have nonspecific complaints such as viral illnesses, joint pain, or fatigue that do not appear to warrant an emergency response. Exam staff members should offer to have the physician speak with an SP who has a particular complaint. If the SP is reluctant or refuses, and there is any question about the health or safety of the SP, staff members should consult the physician for recommendations on how to proceed through the exam.

5.4   Medical Management and Referrals

5.4.1   Medical Referrals

Although the primary purpose of the MEC examination is data collection, not diagnosis or treatment, the exam may produce findings that warrant further medical attention. There is an obligation to inform the SP of any abnormal results from the exams, and to refer the SP to the appropriate provider for treatment. The MEC physician is responsible for the referral process. Each exam component has a referral process built into the ISIS system, which will alert the physician to findings that may require a referral. Some of the exam findings may already be known to the SPs and their providers, but others may have been unknown until the day of the MEC exam. Based on the results of any component of the MEC examination, the physician will place the examinee in one of three categories:

Level I   Major medical findings that warrant immediate attention by a health care provider, e.g., dangerously high blood pressure, emergencies.

Level II   Major medical findings that warrant attention by a health care provider in the next 2 weeks because they are expected to cause adverse effects within this time period.

Level III   Minor medical findings that an examinee and his or her physician already know about. Medical findings that do not require prompt attention by a medical provider.

A Level I referral usually results in termination of the MEC exam, with a transfer of the SP out of the MEC and into a hospital or other care facility. If an SP refuses treatment, she or he must sign a release stating that she or he is aware of the exam findings and is refusing treatment against the advice of the MEC physician. The SP must sign the release form before leaving the MEC.

An SP with a Level II referral can continue the MEC examination and will be advised to see his or her primary care provider within the 2 weeks following the exam. If the SP does not have a care provider, the MEC physician can arrange for the SP to see a local provider who has previously agreed to accept referrals from the MEC exam.

5.4.2   Medical Management

The following section describes some medical scenarios that may occur during the MEC examination and actions to be taken by the MEC physician. The section also provides guidance in determining the level of referral for an examinee.

5.4.2.1   Allergic Reactions

Examinees who experience allergic reactions will be treated according to the procedures adopted from Phil Lieberman, M.D., *Conn's Current Therapy*, 1981, which states: "the therapy of anaphylaxis and anaphylactic reactions is subdivided into those procedures which are to be performed immediately and those which require a more detailed evaluation of the patient prior to transfer to the institution." Procedures that should be instituted immediately are:

1.   The administration of epinephrine is the most important single therapeutic measure. Epinephrine should be administered at the first appearance of symptoms. Early administration can prevent more serious manifestations. The route of administration should be intramuscular or subcutaneous. Intravenous administration should be avoided if possible, being reserved only for those rare instances in which there is loss of consciousness and obvious severe cardiovascular collapse.

     The dose of intramuscular or subcutaneous epinephrine is 0.3 to 0.5ml of a 1:1000 concentration. Injections may be administered every 10 to 15 minutes until an effect is achieved or until tachycardia or other side effects supervene.

     The aforementioned subcutaneous and intramuscular dose is for adults. Children should receive a dose of 0.01 ml per kg of 1:1000 epinephrine to a maximum of 0.3 ml.

2.   The airway should be checked immediately. Laryngeal edema and angioedema of the tissue surrounding the airway is the most rapid cause of death.

3.   The SP should be placed in a recumbent position and his or her feet elevated.

4.   Nasal oxygen should be started.

5.   Vital signs should be obtained and monitored every 10 to 15 minutes for the duration of the attack.

After the procedures noted above have been done, a more extensive evaluation can be performed. The injection of epinephrine may be sufficient to prevent further symptoms. If, however, the SP continues to have difficulty, other measures are instituted as deemed appropriate according to the patient's evaluation.

5.4.2.2   First Aid for Choking

Infants, children, and adults who are choking as a result of a foreign body obstruction should be treated according to the guidelines recommended in basic life support courses.

For adults and children older than 1 year, the Heimlich maneuver is the treatment of choice. A series of six to ten rapid, upward abdominal thrusts can be performed until the foreign body is expelled. If the obstruction is not relieved using the Heimlich maneuver, the victim's airway should be opened using the tongue-jaw lift. If the object can be seen, it can be removed with a finger sweep. If the object cannot be seen, blind finger sweeps can be attempted on adults. Blind finger sweeps can cause further airway obstruction, however, and should never be done on children.

For choking infants, place the infant face down on the rescuer's forearm in a 60-degree head-down position with the head and neck stabilized. A series of back blows and chest thrusts should be performed until the airway obstruction is relieved.

For further information on treatment of choking victims, both conscious and unconscious, consult the *Emergency Medicine Manual*.

5.4.2.3   Seizures

Examinees who experience a seizure while in the MEC should receive immediate attention from the physician. The following steps should be taken to secure the safety of the examinee:

Step 1.   Position the examinee on the ground.

Step 2.   Insert an oral airway if the jaw is relaxed. (Do not **force** any object into the mouth.)

Step 3.   Remove glasses and loosen collar.

Step 4.   Remove objects from vicinity of examinee to prevent injury.

Step 5.   Monitor vital signs.

The MEC physician must use his or her clinical judgment based on the examinee's past medical history, the type and duration of the seizure, the cause of the seizure, and current seizure medication to determine whether or not the person needs emergency medical care or can be sent home. The MEC physician is also responsible for maintaining an airway, giving any indicated medications, and directing care of a seizing examinee until an ambulance arrives or the seizure is over.

5.4.2.4   Hypoglycemia

Most conditions of hypoglycemia can be treated while the subject is conscious with the simple administration of juice and other first aid measures. If hypoglycemia is suspected in the case of an unconscious examinee, the following steps may be taken after emergency assistance is summoned:

Step 1. Recognition of hypoglycemia based on available history:

- Bizarre behavior and other clinical signs of possible glucose insufficiency should lead the physician to think of hypoglycemia. Hypoglycemia may develop in both diabetic and nondiabetic individuals.

Step 2. Basic life support:

- Immediate management includes positioning (supine), airway maintenance, oxygen administration, and monitoring of vital signs. The hypoglycemic examinee will not regain consciousness until the blood glucose level is elevated.

Step 3. Definitive management:

- An unconscious person with a prior history of diabetes mellitus is always presumed to be hypoglycemic unless other causes of unconsciousness are present. Definitive management of the unconscious diabetic usually entails the administration of a carbohydrate by the most effective route available. The most effective route is usually intravenous administration of 50 percent dextrose solution. The unconscious examinee must **never** be given anything by mouth, since this may add to the possibility of airway obstruction or pulmonary aspiration. In the absence of intravenous fluids, definitive management must await the arrival of local emergency assistance.

5.4.2.5   Use of Oxygen

When the oxygen tank is used in the MEC, the flow rate should be set between 3-6 liters/minute unless the person has Chronic Obstructive Pulmonary Disease (COPD). With the use of the nasal cannula, a flow range of 3-6 liters/minute produces a forced inspiratory oxygen of 40 to 50 percent. If the SP self-reported COPD, the flow rate should be set at 2 liters per minute. At this rate, there is little to no danger of interfering with the hypoxic-breathing stimulus present in COPD.

5.5   Emergency Procedures

5.5.1   Medical Emergencies Overview

Before examinations begin at a stand, the facility and equipment specialist (FES) will have obtained information from the advance team about the types and availability of emergency medical services in the area where the MEC is located. The FES will also invite the emergency medical service to tour the MEC prior to the start day of SP examinations. Emergency medical services can include those available at nearby hospitals, hospital ambulance services, and emergency services available from police and fire rescue squads as well as from other county or local rescue squads. The phone number "911" is to be used if applicable for the MEC location. However, the telephone numbers of the nearest police, fire, and rescue squads will also be posted. Execution of emergency procedures and the proper use of all emergency equipment will be the responsibility of the MEC physician. The primary response of the MEC physician should be to stabilize the examinee's condition and to expedite a safe transfer to the nearest emergency medical treatment facility.

The MEC examinations are designed to be safe for examinees. To ensure maximal safety, the physician must be able to handle the initial management of an examinee in distress.

The response of the physician is limited by a number of factors. There are no nurses, respiratory therapists, physician's assistants, or other specialized staff that are necessary for a high-level emergency response. The MEC is not a diagnostic or treatment center, and the liability insurance obtained for Westat physicians does not cover any type of treatment procedure (except emergency stabilization). Within these restrictions, the appropriate response of the physician should be, as previously stated, to stabilize the examinee in distress and facilitate a safe and expedited transfer to the nearest medical facility.

The physician is responsible for directing the care of a patient in the event of an emergency. Staff members are responsible for the tasks assigned to them under the direction of the MEC manager and the physician.

The best overall approach to medical emergencies is prevention. The physician may be called upon to decide if some procedures should not be administered to certain examinees to avoid potential medical problems if the examinee does not fit easily into the preexisting medical exclusion categories for that procedure. The examining physician can at his or her discretion proscribe certain procedures such as respiratory health and other tests if he or she believes the test may endanger an examinee's health. The specific reasons for excluding the examinee should be recorded in the system in the comment drop-down list.

Standard first aid approaches are to be followed for common problems such as faints, minor seizures, falls, and other minor injuries. The MEC physician will determine the level of treatment and referral based on the circumstances of each case. Caution should be exercised and there should be no hesitation to send an examinee to an emergency room when circumstances warrant.

The physician is to be notified immediately of any situation involving an examinee whose safety is of concern. Any questionable situation should be considered an emergency and evaluated by the physician. In addition to the equipment and supplies that are transported to the site at the time of the emergency, a list of the medications (prescription and nonprescription) that the examinee is currently taking will be available. The medication list may provide pertinent medical history information to the physician so that a more accurate assessment of the examinee can be made and the appropriate emergency treatment given. The medication list is the one obtained by the interviewer in the household questionnaire, and is available in the Physician's Exam ISIS application.

When ambulance personnel trained in emergency medical care arrive to transport an examinee in distress (Level I referral), the physician should make an assessment of whether he or she should accompany the examinee to the emergency room. The decision should be based on maximizing safety for the examinee. If the physician determines that he or she should accompany the examinee to the hospital, the MEC must be closed. The field office will contact the examinee's family as soon as possible to inform them of the incident and the medical facility to which the examinee was taken. The physician may also contact the examinee's designated primary health care providers as soon as possible to inform them of the occurrence and the name of the medical facility to which the examinee was taken.

5.5.1.1   Emergency Supplies and Equipment

A limited number of emergency supplies are located in the physician's room, described below.

Emergency cardiac and respiratory care supplies located in the physician room:

- Oxygen tanks (2)
  - Primary: Secured to wall beside window
  - Backup: Secured to wall under desk
- Oxygen masks and tubing (kept in oxygen tank carrying case)
  - Nasal Canula: 1 adult, 1 pediatric
  - Oxygen Mask: 1 mask
  - Extension Tubing
- Automatic External Defibrillator
- Emergency Kit - medications
  - Albuterol
  - Ammonia Ampules
  - Aspirin, 325 mg tablets
  - Diphenhydramine liquid 12.5 mg/5ml
  - Diphenhydramine tablets 25mg
  - Epi Pen – Adult
  - Epi Pen – Junior

- Glucose Tube

- Nitrostat

■ Emergency Kit – supplies

- Spare AED Battery

- Pocket BP cuffs – child, adult, and large adult

- Stethoscope (2) child and adult

- Protective eyewear

- Tongue depressor

- Scissors

- Pen light

- Sterile gloves - Two pairs

- ½" Transpore tape

- Surgilube packets

- Oral airways: infant, small, medium, large

The drugs in the emergency kit are described in more detail in Table 5–1.

Table 5–1.   Drugs in emergency kit

Medication	Form supplied	Dose	Route administered
Albuterol (17g)	Metered dose canister	90 mcg/puff	Inhaled
Ammonia	Ammonia Aspirol	0.3 ml	Inhaled
Aspirin	Unit dose package	325 mg	Oral
Diphenhydramine	Liquid	12.5mg/5ml	Oral
Diphenhydramine	Tablets	25mg	Oral
Epinephrine-adult	EpiPen	0.3 mg 1:1000	IM injection
Epinephrine-peds	EpiPen Jr.	0.15 mg 1:2000	IM injection
Glucose – tube	Insta-Glucose 31 gm	1-2 tbsp	Oral
Nitroglycerin (25 tabs)	Nitrostat	0.4mg 1/150gr	Sublingual

Please note that the drug kit does not contain antiarrythmic medications or narcotics. Only the physician should administer emergency procedures and use the contents of the emergency supplies other than the stethoscope and blood pressure cuff.

Oxygen Cylinders and Supplies

There are two size D aluminum oxygen cylinders on the mobile examination center. The cylinders are 15.27" long by 4.38" diameter with an oxygen capacity of 415 liters. The **PRIMARY** oxygen cylinder is attached to the wall beside the window. The regulator must be attached at all times. The cylinder and regulator are encased in a soft nylon padded carrying bag with a shoulder strap for ease of carrying it during an emergency. Oxygen administration supplies are stored in the external pockets of the bag. The physician is responsible for conducting an inventory of all oxygen administration supplies at stand setup and teardown, and ordering replacements through the inventory management system.

The **BACKUP** oxygen cylinder is secured to the wall under the desk in the physician's room. This cylinder and regulator are also encased inside a soft carry bag. When the primary cylinder is off the MEC, the backup cylinder should be moved to the primary cylinder location until the primary cylinder is returned. The oxygen administration supplies should remain on the MEC at all times.

Oxygen Administration

The primary oxygen cylinder should be used first in all emergencies. If oxygen is depleted from this cylinder, then the backup cylinder should be used. A full cylinder will vary in clinically effective usage time, but an estimate of usage time is approximately 25 minutes when running at 8L/min.

Oxygen is regarded as a medication and should be administered only by or with the direction of a qualified health care provider. On the MEC, the physician is the staff member designated to determine the necessity of oxygen administration, and will provide other MEC staff with instructions regarding method of administration and the flow rate. Whenever oxygen is administered *for any length of time,* the physician is responsible for recording all information regarding the oxygen administration on the Oxygen Usage Log (Attached, Oxygen Usage and Record Form). Any administration of oxygen constitutes an emergency or incident, and the physician must also complete the emergency forms on the MEC.

The backup oxygen cylinder should be used for all instructional and training purposes. The primary cylinder should never be used for this purpose.

Oxygen Cylinder Monitoring

The MEC manager and the physician are responsible for monitoring the supply of oxygen for both the primary and the backup cylinders. The regulator readings should be recorded on the **Oxygen Cylinder Monitoring Log** at the following times throughout each stand: on setup day, **every Monday** during the afternoon or evening session, and at teardown. If the team is not working on Monday, then the supply level should be checked during the next session worked. Both the MEC manager and the physician are responsible for signing the form when the oxygen level is checked. The completed forms are sent to the home office at the end of the stand with all other end of stand mailings.

Oxygen Tank Refilling/Replacement

When either cylinder is less than one–half full, the facility and equipment specialist is responsible for refilling the cylinder. During SP sessions, one cylinder must be present on the MEC, even if only half full. Never remove both cylinders for refilling at the same time during the stand when SPs will be present. NCHS provides Westat with a prescription letter to be kept with the FES, and a copy of the letter will be retained at the Westat home office. Oxygen suppliers almost always require a prescription for oxygen; however, this depends on the laws of individual states. At this time, we do not switch out the cylinder, as is the practice with most oxygen replenishment practices—the cylinders on the MECs are refilled so that we can provide standardization of the regulators and tanks as the MEC travels across the country.

Automated External Defibrillator

The automated external defibrillator (AED) requires one battery to function during use. The par level for defibrillator batteries on each MEC is 2. This par level assures that if the primary battery fails, becomes outdated, or is totally discharged during use, that there will be a backup battery for the AED. The expiration date for each battery is set by the manufacturer and is recorded on the battery, as well as on the Physician Examination start of stand and end of stand inventory forms. The importance of assuring the availability of these critical inventory items cannot be overemphasized. This is a start of stand, weekly, mid stand, and end of stand QC check requirement.

Reference Materials in the Physician Exam Room

Reference materials available to the physician include:

1. *The Merck Manual of Diagnosis and Therapy*, 18th Edition. Mark H. Beer, Robert S. Porter, Thomas V. Jones. April 2006. Wiley Publishers.

2. *Physician's Desk Reference 2008*; Thompson Healthcare.

3. *Emergency Medicine Manual*, 6th Edition. O. John Ma, David M. Cline, Judith E. Tintinalli, Gabor D. Kelen, J. Stephan Stapczynski 2004, McGraw-Hill Companies, Inc.

5.5.1.2   MEC Standard Medical Emergency Protocol

Due to the limited space in the MEC trailers, congregations of more than three or four people in one room are almost impossible. Subsequently, staff response to an emergency has been designed to limit the number of people needed to be together at one time. For example, a true cardiac or respiratory arrest requires only three people to be close to the patient for an extended period of time: two staff members to perform CPR and one physician. Two staff members will act as a runner and a recorder, but will be required to do so without hindering the performance of CPR or the physician's access to the patient. Once an ambulance arrives, the path to the victim must be clear to allow transfer to Emergency Medical Services (EMS) staff. If possible, the closest emergency exit door should be opened for EMS personnel to transfer the patient to an ambulance. Other types of emergencies, such as a fall or a seizure, will require the presence of the physician and only one or two staff as requested by the physician and the MEC manager. There should be no spectators in the vicinity that may inhibit care of a patient.

5.5.1.3   Staff Roles in an Emergency

First Responder

The first responder is the person who either discovers the victim or is with the victim at the time of the event. Do not leave the victim alone at any time. Call for another staff member to alert the coordinator and the physician of the situation immediately and initiate CPR if needed. The first person who responds to your call will be the runner for the event. If another staff member is immediately available, call for that person to assist you with CPR. If no one is available, continue one-person CPR until someone arrives to assist you. Once the physician arrives, explain briefly what happened and she or he will direct care of the patient while you and your partner continue CPR. The physician will also ensure that there is a designated recorder for the event.

If the physician is the first person on the scene, she or he should call for help to alert the coordinator and MEC manager immediately and then initiate CPR if needed. The physician should continue one-person CPR until two other staff members arrive to take over CPR while the physician directs care of the patient. The MEC manager will confirm that all roles in the emergency response have been filled, and that all unneeded staff are clear of the area. If the coordinator has taken on a role in the emergency, the MEC manager will assign another staff member to take over for the coordinator. The coordinator will then return to the reception area to manage the SPs in the MEC. If the MEC manager is not in the MEC at the time of the event, the chief health technologist should be notified to follow the MEC manager's emergency protocol responsibilities.

Laboratory Staff

1.   Activate the Emergency Medical Services (EMS) system by calling 911 or other emergency numbers posted at the coordinator station. Request an ambulance for a medical emergency and give the location of the MEC.

Coordinator

The coordinator's responsibilities in the event of an emergency are as follows:

1.   Notify the MEC manager of the emergency and provide any information you have regarding the need for staff assignments. If the MEC manager is not in the MEC at the time of the event, notify the chief health technologist who will then follow the MEC manager's emergency protocol responsibilities.

2.   Retrieve any SPs left unattended in exam rooms while staff members are assisting with the emergency. Staff should remain in the exam rooms with the SPs if they are not called upon to assist in the emergency. All other SPs should remain in the reception area with the coordinator. If the event occurs in the reception area, SPs in the reception area should be escorted to other exam rooms.

3.   Remain in the reception area with the SPs or designate another staff member to do so. Maintain calm and assure SPs the situation is under control.

MEC Manager

The MEC manager's responsibilities in the event of an emergency are as follows:

1.   Check that the following response team is on the scene: 1 runner, 1 recorder, 2 people performing CPR (if necessary), and the physician.

2.   Check that all other staff members are clear of the area.

3.   Post the assistant coordinator or other available staff member outside the MEC to direct EMS to the site of the emergency.

4.   Locate the emergency exit closest to the site of the emergency to facilitate transfer of the patient to EMS. The cargo lift on trailer 2 is **NOT** approved for transporting SPs from the MEC.

5.   Contact the field office immediately after the SP has left the MEC to inform the field office manager of the emergency. The field office will notify the SP's family of the event if the SP came alone to the MEC.

If the MEC manager is not available at the time of the emergency, the chief health technologist will follow the protocol for the MEC manager's responsibilities.

Assistant Coordinator

The assistant coordinator, when available, will be stationed outside the entrance to the MEC and will direct EMS into the MEC and to the site of the emergency. If an emergency exit door has been opened, the assistant coordinator will direct EMS to the emergency exit door to facilitate transfer of the victim. If the assistant coordinator is not available, another staff member can be designated to guide the EMS team.

MEC Physician

The MEC physician is responsible for directing care of the SP until EMS arrives. Once the emergency equipment is on the scene, the physician should ensure that a staff member is recording events on the MEC Incident/Emergency Report form. The physician should not perform tasks such as CPR unless he or she is the first person on the scene. If the physician is the first responder, she or he should begin CPR until two other staff members arrive. The physician is also responsible for the operation of the automated external defibrillator and the administration of medications. The physician will follow the ACLS algorithm and emergency protocols as outlined in the physician manual. When ambulance personnel trained in emergency medical care arrive to transport an SP in distress (Level I referral), the physician should make an assessment of whether she or he should accompany the SP to the emergency room. The decision whether or not to provide an escort to the hospital should be based on maximizing safety for the SP. If the physician determines that she or he should accompany the SP to the hospital, the MEC must be closed. If possible, the physician should obtain consent from the SP or the SP's family to contact the SP's designated primary health care provider as soon as possible to report the occurrence and give the name of the medical facility to which the SP was taken.

Recorder

Any staff member could be called upon to act as recorder for the event. The recorder will be responsible for documenting the time of the emergency and the sequence of events that follow the initiation of emergency care on the MEC Incident/Emergency Report form (Exhibit 5-3).[*] The order of the events and time sequence are the critical elements in documentation. MEC Incident/Emergency Report forms will be kept in the physician's emergency kit and are available on ISIS by clicking on the ambulance icon in the Toolbox. Instructions for completing this form are found in Exhibit 5-4 of this manual.

Runner

Generally, the first person to respond to the call for help will be the runner for the event. The runner's first responsibility is to notify the physician, the coordinator, and the MEC manager of the event. Once the appropriate people have been notified, the runner is responsible for retrieving supplies and equipment and making phone calls as directed by staff at the scene.

Other staff members should remain clear of the site and assist in keeping order in the MEC unless asked to help. No SPs should be left alone in the MEC. If a staff member has a role in the emergency and is in the process of examining an SP, the SP will be returned to the reception area while the staff member is in the emergency. All other staff will remain in the exam rooms with SPs until the crisis has passed. The coordinator is responsible for managing SPs in the reception area. The MEC manager is responsible for managing the MEC staff. In the absence of the MEC manager, the chief technologist will manage the MEC staff response during the emergency.

5.5.1.4 The Physician's Role and AED Operation

As explained previously, the MEC is not a diagnostic or treatment center, and the liability insurance obtained for Westat physicians does not cover any type of treatment procedure (except emergency stabilization). The primary response of the MEC physician should be to stabilize the

---

[*] All exhibits are located at the end of this chapter.

examinee's condition and to expedite a safe transfer to the nearest emergency medical treatment facility. MEC physicians are required to be BLS certified. The physician is the only person responsible for the operation of the AED, and the administration of oxygen and medications (Exhibit 5-1). The AED can be placed on a patient for the purpose of monitoring a heart rhythm, but only one lead will be displayed. The physician is not expected to make a diagnosis based on the AED monitor. The AED should be used only for monitoring a heart rate, or when ventricular tachycardia or ventricular fibrillation is suspected or imminent. Any patient who is unconscious is a candidate for application of the AED. The AED will advise a shock only in the event of ventricular tachycardia or fibrillation. The AED does not have cardioversion capability, nor will the physician be able to deliver a shock if the AED does not advise a shock. As there are no antiarrythmic medications in the emergency drug kit, the response to a cardiac emergency is basic life support with defibrillation if indicated.

5.5.1.5   Documentation

After the SP has left the MEC, the physician should make sure that the incident and outcome are documented in the automated system in the physician's ISIS application. The physician will also complete a full report on a separate form, the MEC Incident/Emergency Report form, described below. The recorder will also use this form to record events on the scene. The recorder's notes of the event will be especially important in the completion of the physician's report and should be kept with the physician's documentation of the incident. The MEC manager should review the final report prepared by the physician and add any information not included in the physician's report. The MEC manager's addendum should include only information about the event that is not in the physician's report. Any discrepancies in reports should be brought to the attention of the Director of MEC Operations before being made final. Notification and documentation of the emergency incident should be directed to Catherine Novak, Director of MEC Operations, as soon as possible.

5.5.1.6   MEC Incident/Emergency Report Form

A hard-copy form titled "MEC Incident/Emergency Report" will be used for recording the sequence of events or actions that are taken during the emergency response. An example of the form is shown in Exhibit 5-3. Guidelines for completion of the form are in Exhibit 5-4. During the emergency, the recorder will use the form to record vitals, treatments, and some patient outcomes. The physician will then use the recorder's notes to complete a final official MEC Incident/Emergency Report form. The MEC manager will then review the final form with the physician and make any necessary additions.

The NHANES Emergency Protocol Checklist (Exhibit 5-2), and the MEC Incident/Emergency Report Form Documentation Guidelines (Exhibit 5-4) are located in the emergency kit in the physician's exam room. The NHANES Emergency Protocol Checklist is also located in the major hallways of the MEC.

5.6   Psychiatric/Behavioral Problem Procedures

There are situations that may arise regarding SP behavior that will require special handling. They include:

- Previous psychological injuries, deterioration, and/or deprivation – Due to changes in mental status, the SP may seem confused or may actually have dementia.

- Inebriation due to intoxication with alcohol and/or drugs – The SP will be less able to grasp ideas, reason, problem solve, calculate, and attend to the tasks at hand. Therefore, the potential for injury, trauma, and violence is present.

- Belligerence – This will include SPs with noncompliant or abusive behavior.

- Suicidal/Homicidal Ideation – If an SP expresses intent to harm him/herself or someone else, the SP should be referred to the physician. The physician will evaluate the SP and determine the need for a referral to a psychiatric facility.

If the SP is so demented, confused, intoxicated, or belligerent that it is impossible to continue the examination, the MEC manager should calmly terminate the MEC examination and have the examinee leave the center without delay. For those examinees who require assistance going home, have a family member escort them home or call a cab.

Suicidal and homicidal ideation are considered psychiatric emergencies and are generally handled by referral.

For any psychiatric emergency, an incident form should be completed and the incident reported by telephone to the Director of MEC Operations as soon as possible.

5.7 Natural Disaster Procedures

In the event of an unforeseeable occurrence (i.e., hurricane, tornado, fire, etc.), certain procedures should be followed depending on whether the event happens before or during an examination session.

5.7.1 Disaster Prior to an Examination Session (Predicted Event)

- The stand coordinator should contact the home office for instructions regarding whether to cancel the session. If the session is canceled, the stand coordinator will then notify the MEC manager who in turn will notify the MEC staff.

- If residents of mobile homes and trailers have been notified to evacuate, the stand coordinator should make the decision to cancel the session. She or he should then call the home office to report the occurrence and cancellation of the session and notify the MEC manager. The MEC manager should notify the MEC staff.

- The stand coordinator and MEC manager may place the staff on standby procedures, with instructions to be ready to work but accessible by phone at home awaiting orders from the MEC manager regarding status of operations.

5.7.2 Disaster During an Examination Session

If an examination session is underway and SPs are in the MEC when the MEC manager or coordinator is notified by the field office of a pending natural event, the following procedures should be followed:

- The MEC manager and the physician should make a joint decision regarding closing the MEC and/or canceling the session. The first priority should be the safety of the SPs and staff.

- The MEC staff and SPs should evacuate the MEC as soon as possible and go directly to a safe haven, such as a building close by or the staff hotel. The staff and SPs should remain at this site until the impending event is over and it is safe to proceed outside.

- After the event, the MEC manager and the physician should decide whether or not to continue the exam session if the SPs are willing to stay for the rest of the session.

- If either the decision is made to cancel the session or the SPs decline to remain, the appointments for those SPs will need to be rescheduled by the field office.

- It is essential for the MEC manager to notify the stand coordinator of the outcome of events. The stand coordinator should then notify the home office immediately.

- Examiners who were conducting an exam or interview when evacuation of the MEC was ordered should interrupt the exam in the ISIS system. The reason for interruption of the exam must be accurately documented in ISIS and in room logs as soon as possible after the MEC is reopened.

- The MEC coordinator should document the reason for exam components omitted because of the closure of the MEC.

- Staff not requested to be involved in the emergency must stay away from the scene, remain in the exam rooms with SPs, and assist in maintaining order in the MEC.

Exhibit 5-1. AED Algorithm

Automated External Defibrillation (AED) Treatment Algorithm
Emergency cardiac care pending arrival of EMS personnel

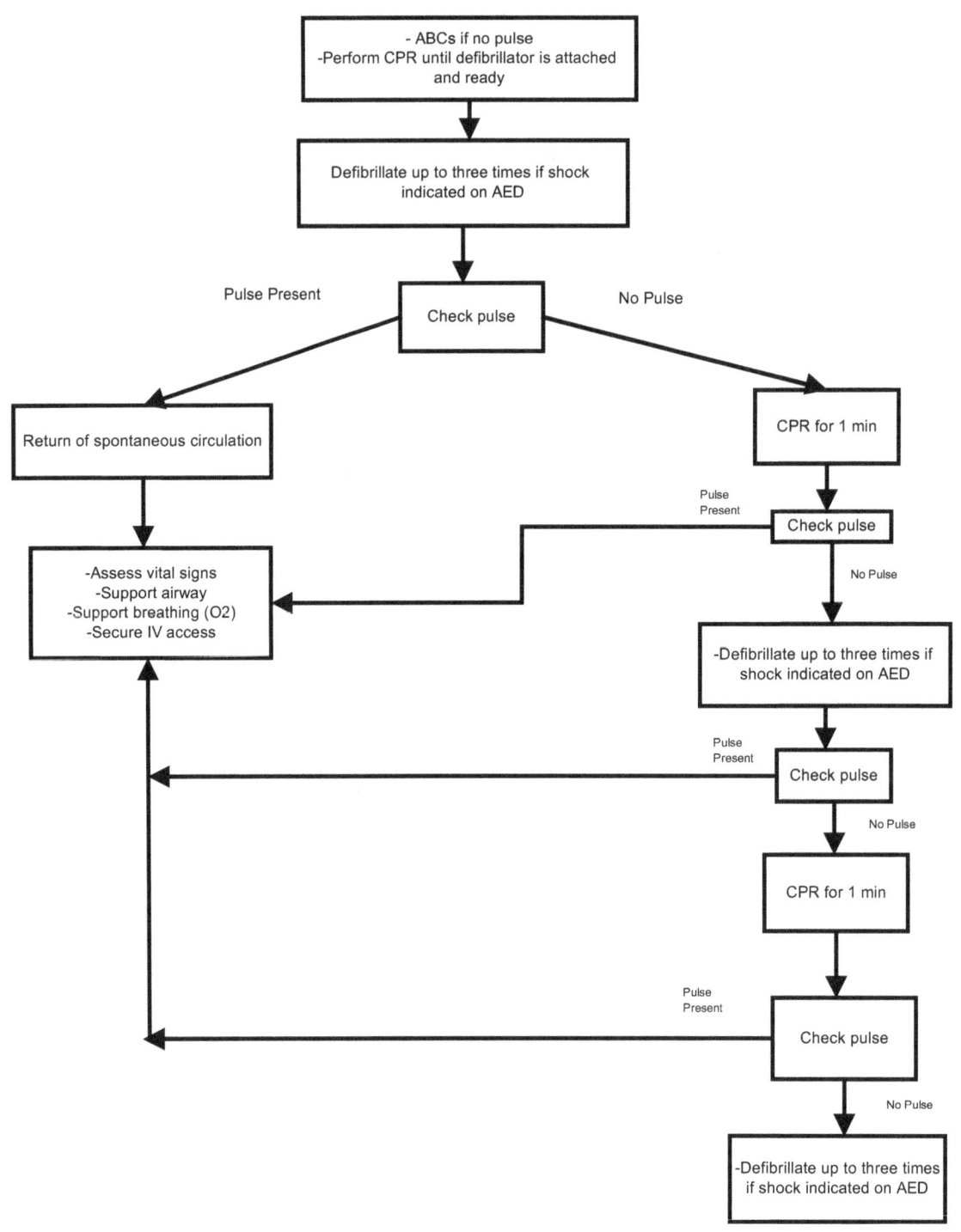

Exhibit 5-2. NHANES Emergency Protocol Checklist

Mobile Examination Center Emergency Management Protocol	
First Responder	✓ Call for help and assess victim for A-B-C, and initiate CPR
	✓ Send closest staff to notify physician, MEC manager, and coordinator of the emergency; this person assumes the role of runner
Physician:	✓ Direct the care of victim until EMS arrives
	✓ Operate automated external defibrillator
	✓ Give medications
	✓ Instruct recorder what to document
Lab Staff	✓ Activate EMS by calling 911 when advised
Coordinator:	✓ Retrieve unattended SPs and return them to the reception area
	✓ Remain with SPs in reception area and provide reassurance
	✓ Confer with MEC manager regarding the continuation of exams
MEC manager: *In the absence of the MEC manager, the Chief Health Tech will assume this role.*	✓ Ensure appropriate number of staff for emergency response; assign as necessary
	✓ Traffic control
	✓ Ensure clear access to the emergency exit door closest to the scene
	✓ Post assistant coordinator or other staff member outside the MEC to greet ambulance personnel
	✓ Notify the field office of the event as soon as possible
Runner:	✓ Obtain equipment and supplies as directed
Recorder:	✓ Record events on the MEC Emergency/Incident Report Form as directed by physician
Assistant coordinator:	✓ Posted at the door to direct ambulance personnel to emergency site

Exhibit 5-3. MEC Incident/Emergency Report form

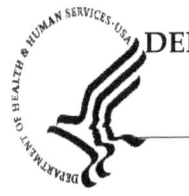 **DEPARTMENT OF HEALTH & HUMAN SERVICES**

Public Health Service
Centers for Disease Control and Prevention

National Center for Health Statistics
6525 Belcrest Road
Hyattsville, Maryland 20782

MEC INCIDENT/EMERGENCY REPORT

Incident/Emergency

◯ Incident   ◯ Emergency

Person Type

◯ SP   ◯ Tech   ◯ Other

General Information

Physician Name:	Recorder Name:
Emergency Date:	Runner Name(s):
Start Time: End Time:	Who Called 911:
Location:	Who Found:
Description:	

Personal Information

Person ID:	Age:	Gender:
Last Name:	First Name:	Middle Name:

DEPARTMENT OF HEALTH & HUMAN SERVICES

Exhibit 5-3. MEC Incident/Emergency Report form (continued)

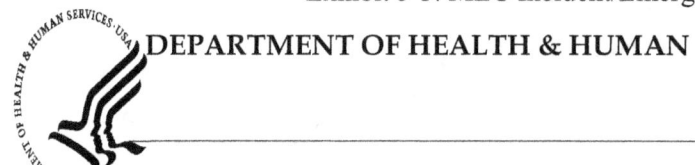

DEPARTMENT OF HEALTH & HUMAN SERVICES

Public Health Service
Centers for Disease Control and Prevention

National Center for Health Statistics
6525 Belcrest Road
Hyattsville, Maryland 20782

Vitals

Time	Heart Rate	Systolic BP	Diastolic BP	Respiratory Rate	Comments

Treatment

Time	Medication/Equipment	Comment

Page 2 of 5

Exhibit 5-3. MEC Incident/Emergency Report form (continued)

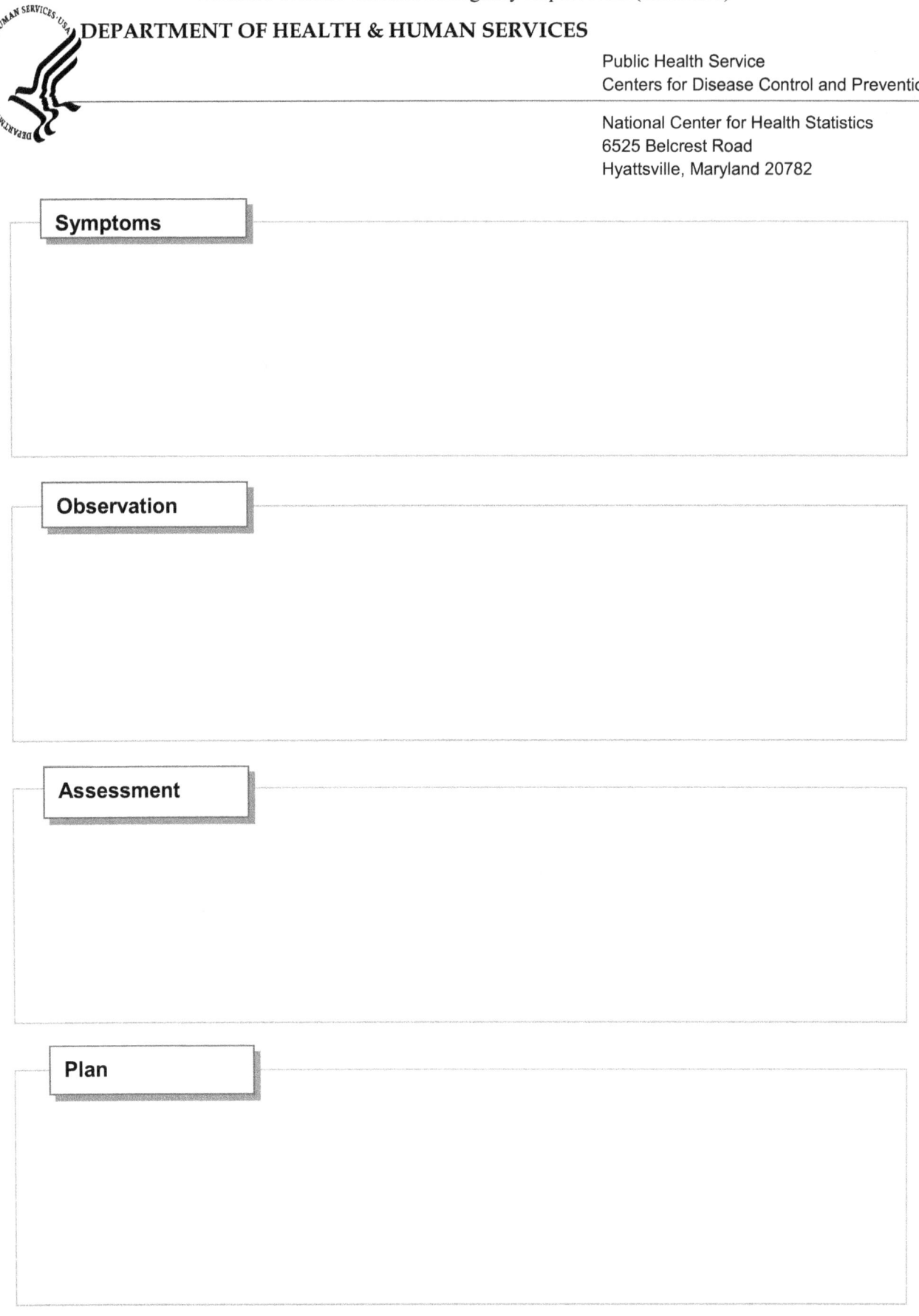

DEPARTMENT OF HEALTH & HUMAN SERVICES

Public Health Service
Centers for Disease Control and Prevention

National Center for Health Statistics
6525 Belcrest Road
Hyattsville, Maryland 20782

Symptoms

Observation

Assessment

Plan

Exhibit 5-3. MEC Incident/Emergency Report form (continued)

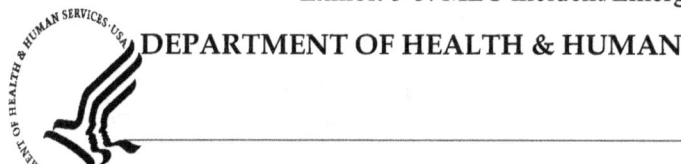

DEPARTMENT OF HEALTH & HUMAN SERVICES

Public Health Service
Centers for Disease Control and Prevention

National Center for Health Statistics
6525 Belcrest Road
Hyattsville, Maryland 20782

Urgent Care

☐ Transported to Hospital	Hospital Name:
Ambulance Arrival Time:	Ambulance Departure Time:
Emergency Service Name:	
☐ Physician Accompanied SP to Hospital	

Notification

☐ Family Member Notified	Name:	Date/time:
	Relation:	
☐ Family Physician Notified	Family Phys Named:	Date/time:

Signature:_____   Date:_____

Exhibit 5-3. MEC Incident/Emergency Report form (continued)

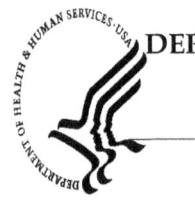

DEPARTMENT OF HEALTH & HUMAN SERVICES

Public Health Service
Centers for Disease Control and Prevention

National Center for Health Statistics
6525 Belcrest Road
Hyattsville, Maryland 20782

Vitals

Time	Heart Rate	Systolic BP	Diastolic BP	Respiratory Rate	Comments

DEPARTMENT OF HEALTH & HUMAN SERVICES   Page 5 of 5

Exhibit 5-4. MEC Incident/Emergency Form Documentation Guidelines

The Vitals and Treatment sections on page 2 should be completed first during the emergency. If the spaces on page 2 are insufficient, the last page should be used for recording vital signs. The "comments" section of the last page can be used to record treatments. The remaining sections should be completed as soon as the emergency is over. The recorder should collect most of the information requested on page 1 before turning the notes over to the physician for compilation of the final report. The following information is to be documented:

Page 1:

- Check either Incident or Emergency, depending on the event. The difference is to be determined by the physician and the MEC manager;

- Check whether the person was an SP, a tech, or other (such as a guest or someone who has accompanied an SP to the exam);

- Names of the physician, runner, recorder, person who called 911, and person who found the victim;

- Date of the emergency response;

- Time that the emergency response started, beginning from the time the victim was found;

- Time that the emergency response ended, i.e., time the ambulance arrived or time the victim left the MEC;

- Location of the emergency in the MEC;

- Description of the victim upon discovery; and

- If the victim is an SP, escort, or guest, the sample number, age, gender, and first and last names should be recorded. If the victim is a staff member, the first and last names are sufficient.

Page 2:

- Vitals and Treatment sections to be recorded at the time of the event by the recorder.

Page 3:

- The sections Symptoms, Observation, Assessment, and Plan are to be completed by the physician after the event.

Exhibit 5-4. MEC Incident/Emergency Form Documentation Guidelines (continued)

Page 4:

- The section Urgent Care is to be completed by the physician if the SP is transported to a hospital;

- The section Notification will be completed by the MEC manager after notifying the field office of the emergency; and

- If the physician has obtained consent from the SP or the SP's family to contact the SP's care provider, the physician must record the name of the physician and the date and time the physician was notified of the SP's status.

6. DOCUMENTATION OF INCIDENTS AND EMERGENCIES

6.1   Incident Forms

If an incident occurs in the MEC, the physician is called to assess the SP. The physician completes an Incident Form as soon as possible after the incident has occurred. Blank Incident/Emergency Report Forms are kept in the emergency kit in the Physician Exam Room. Blank Incident/Emergency Forms may also be printed directly from the ISIS system using the following steps:

- At the Desktop, open Microsoft Word.

- Select "File."

- Select "Open."

- Go to the network drive.

- Select MEC STAFF "H."

- Select "Blank Forms."

- Select "Incident/Emergency Forms."

- A blank form will be opened in "Read-only" mode.

- Select "Print" and click "OK" to print a hard copy of the blank form.

The blank form can be used to temporarily record the details of the incident if it is not convenient to enter the information directly into the system.

At a convenient time, the information is entered directly into the system.

See Exhibit 6-1 for the "Utilities" menu. Exhibit 6-2 is a blank Incident Form. Exhibit 6-3 shows an Incident Form with the vitals completed.

Exhibit 6-1. Utilities menu for Incident/Emergency Form

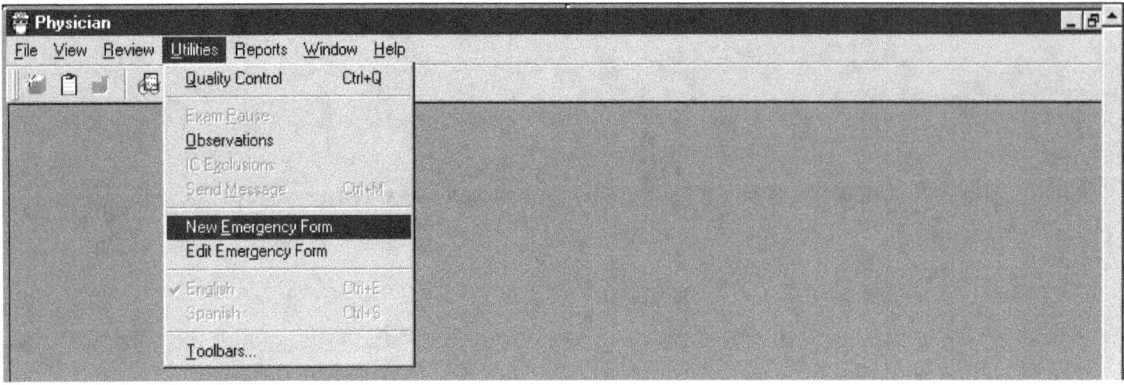

At the "Utilities" menu, select "New Emergency Form" and press "Enter."

Exhibit 6-2. Incident Form – blank

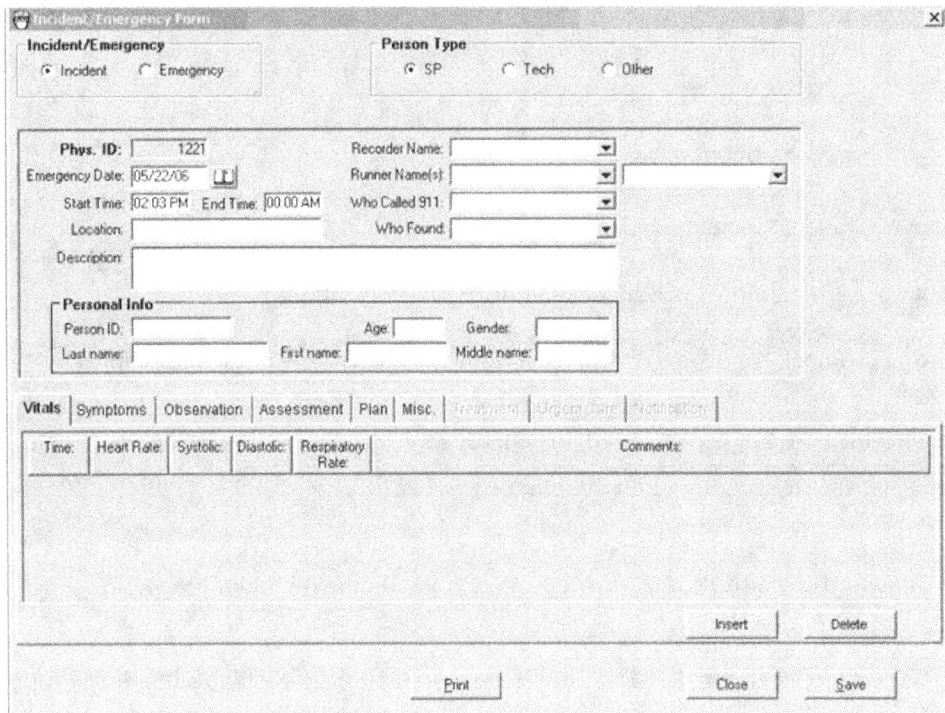

- Select "Incident" or "Emergency" as appropriate.

- Select the "Person Type." The choices are "SP," "Staff," or "Other." "Other" may include visitors or guests.

- The "Date" is automatically entered as the current date. If the incident occurred on an earlier date, the date entered should be the date the incident occurred. The date is a required field.

- The "Start Time" is automatically entered as the time the form was opened. If the incident occurred at an earlier time, the time entered should be the time the incident started. The start time is a required field. Please pay careful attention to this field in order to document the incident/emergency accurately.

- **NOTE:** "AM" is changed to "PM" by pressing "Shift-P" (press the Shift key and the P key) and "PM" is changed to "AM" by pressing "Shift A" (press the Shift key and the "A" key).

- The "End Time" is the time the incident was resolved. This is a required field.

- Enter the location where the incident occurred in the "Location" field.

- Enter a brief description of the incident in the "Description" field.

- Enter the SP's (or staff) ID in the ID field and press the Tab key. The remainder of the "Personal Information" will be automatically entered.

Exhibit 6-3. Incident Form – vitals

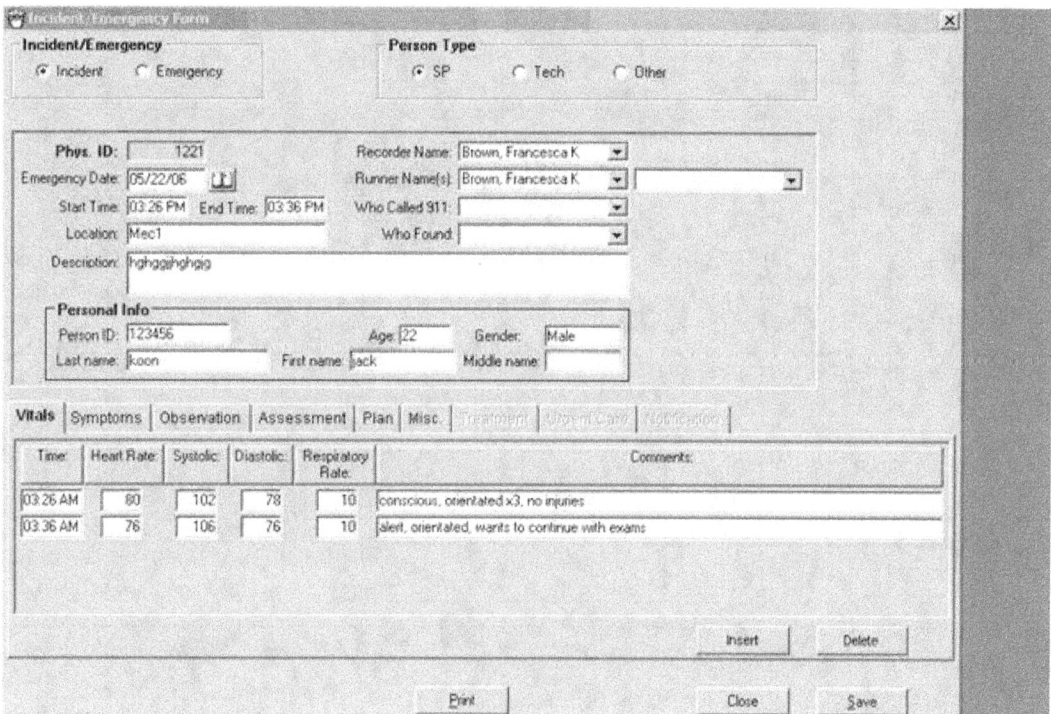

- To add a line to enter "Vitals" information, right click (click the right button on the mouse) and select "Add" or "Insert." This may also be used to delete a line.

- Enter the time the vital signs were taken and then enter the heart rate/minute, systolic and diastolic blood pressure, and respiratory rate/minute.

- Enter a comment to describe the SP's condition at the time the vital signs were taken. Add more lines as necessary.

Click on the Symptoms, Observation, Assessment, Plan, or the miscellaneous (Misc.) tab to open the appropriate field. Information for each of the fields is entered as free text (Exhibit 6-4).

Exhibit 6-4. Incident Form – observations

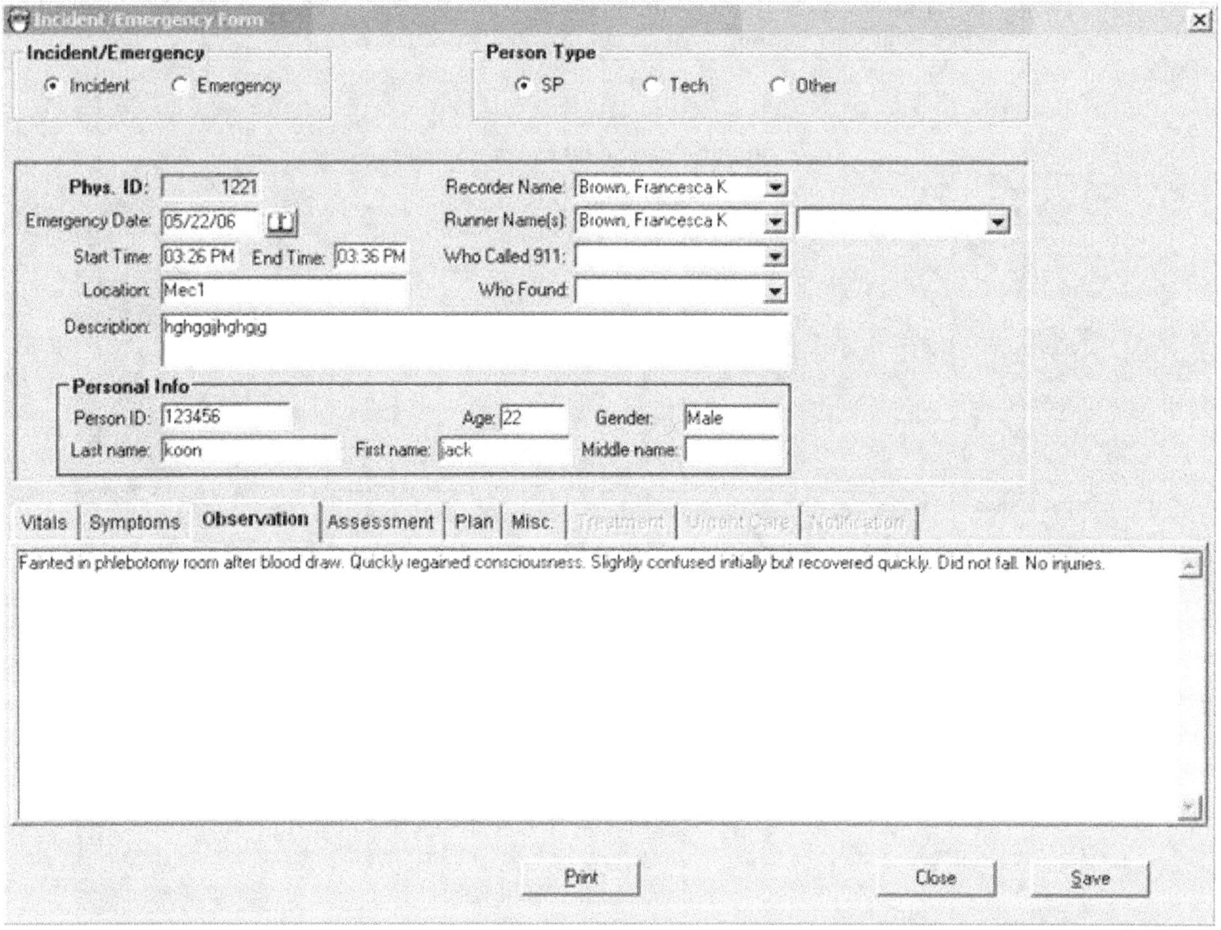

- Select "File" and choose "Save" to close and save the form.

- If you close without saving, a message will be displayed "Do you want to save changes?" (See Exhibit 6-5.)

- Click "Yes" if you want to close and save the form or changes made to the form.

- Click "No" if you want to close without saving the form or changes made to the form.

- Click "Cancel" if you do not want to close the form at this time.

Exhibit 6-5. Incident Form – save

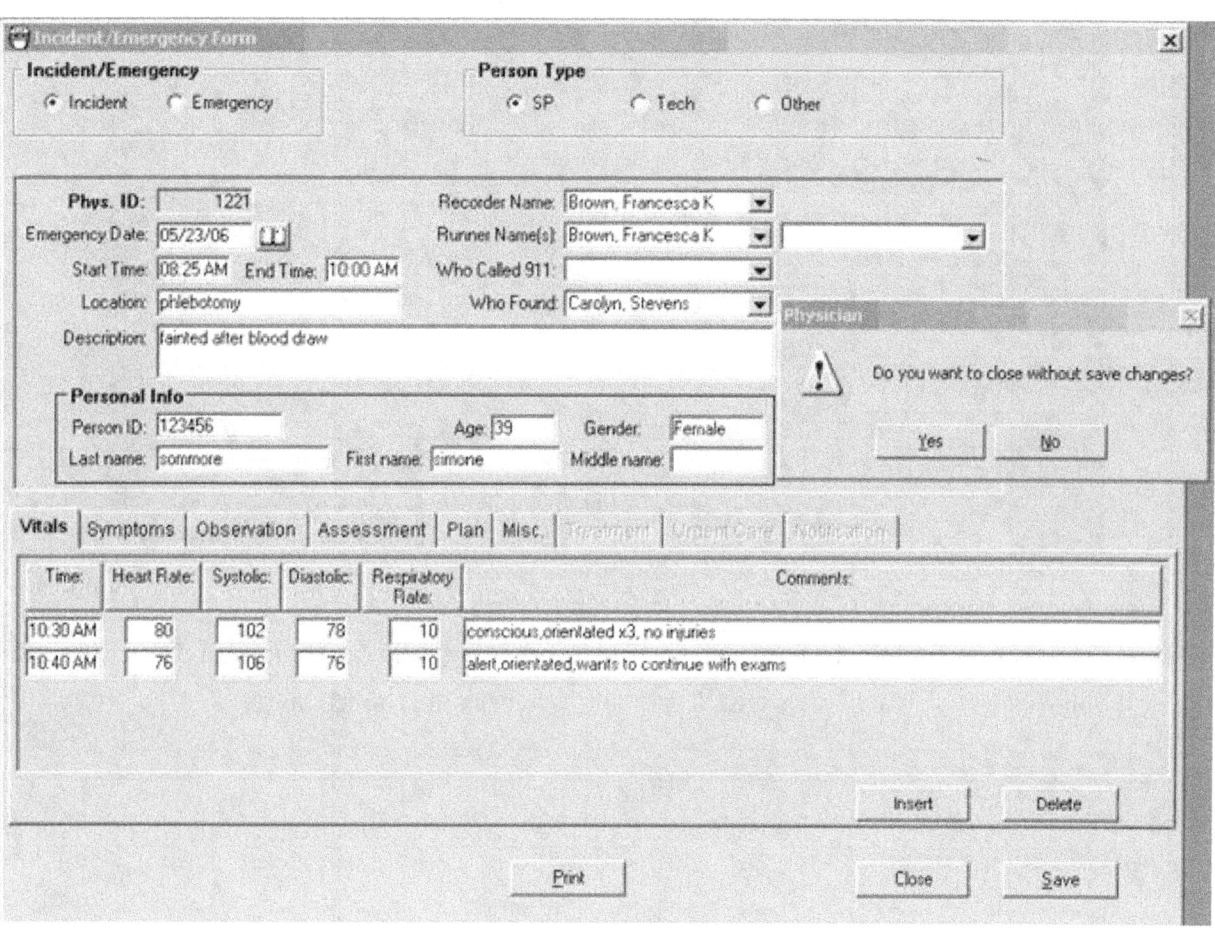

If you try to close the form without entering an "End Time," a message will be displayed "Please enter a valid time." (See Exhibit 6-6.) Click "OK" and enter the time the incident/emergency was completed.

Exhibit 6-6. Incident Form – required fields

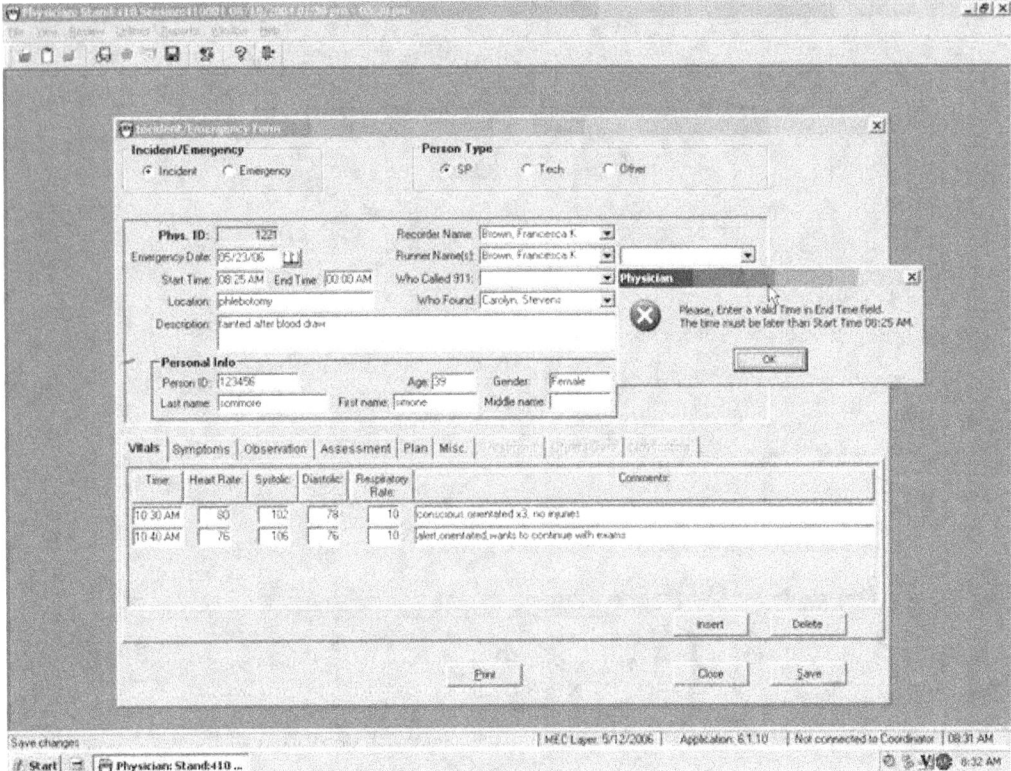

If you try to close the form and the "End Time" is not valid (end time must be later than start time), the above message will be displayed. Click "OK" and enter the correct time.

Exhibit 6-7 shows the tab for "Vitals" for both the Incident and Emergency Forms.

Exhibit 6-7. Incident Form tab marks – vitals

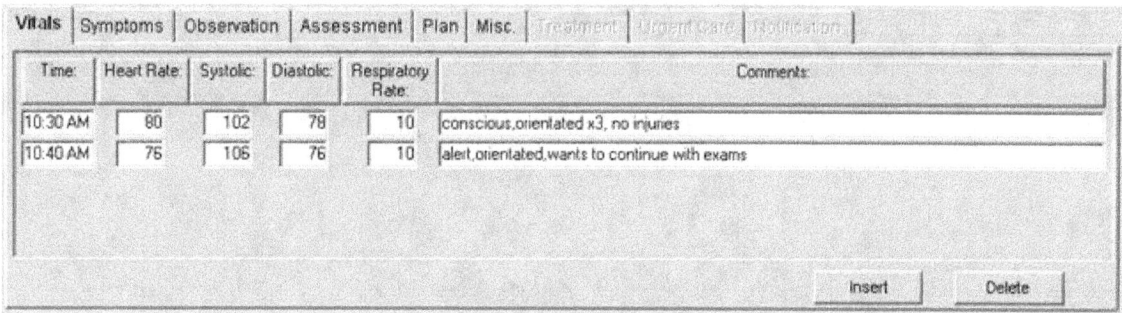

Exhibit 6-8 shows the tab for "Symptoms" for both Incident and Emergency Forms.

Exhibit 6-8. Incident Form – symptoms

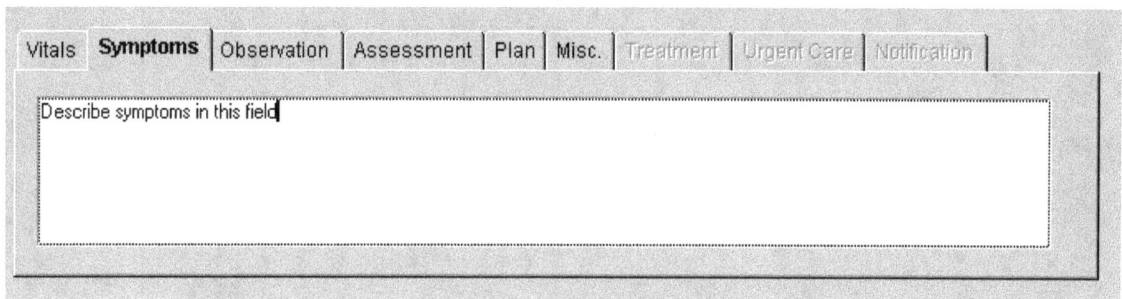

Exhibit 6-9 shows the tab for "Observations" for both Incident and Emergency Forms.

Exhibit 6-9. Incident Form – observation

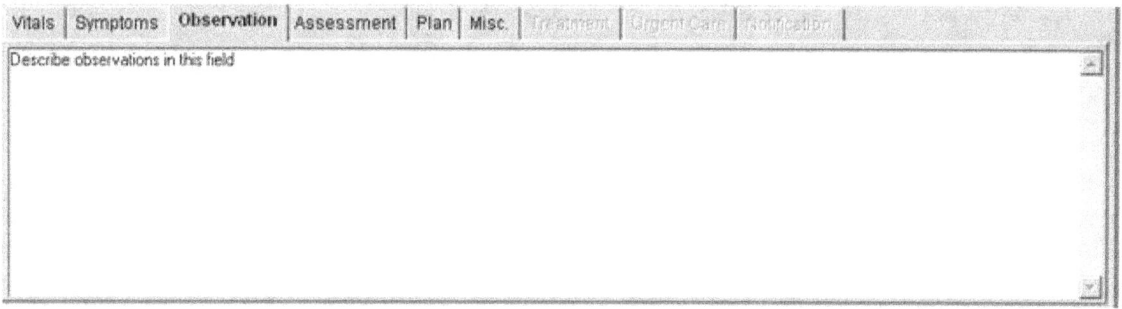

Exhibit 6-10 shows the tab for "Assessment" for both Incident and Emergency Forms.

Exhibit 6-10. Incident Form – assessment

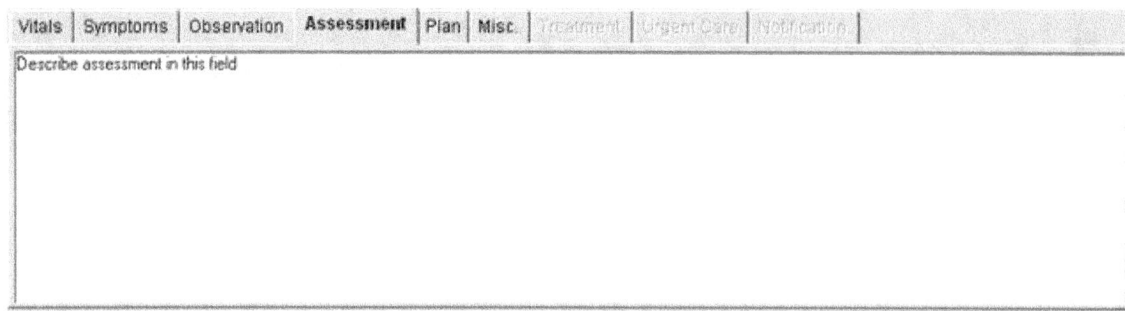

Exhibit 6-11 shows the tab for "Plan" for both Incident and Emergency Forms.

Exhibit 6-11. Incident Form – plan

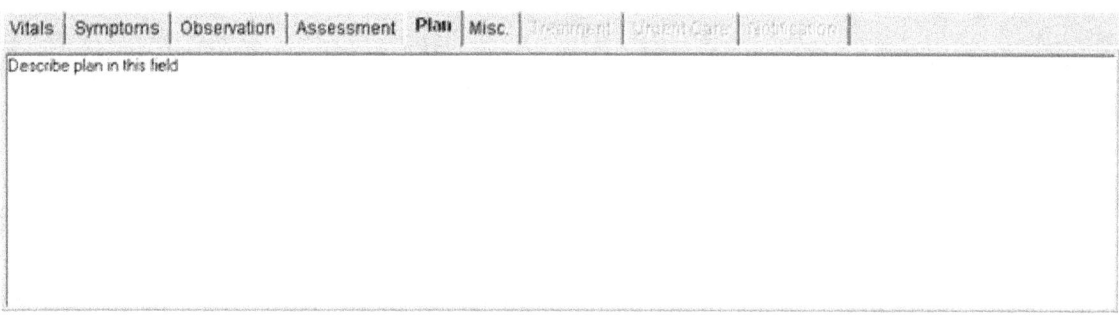

Exhibit 6-12 shows the tab for "Miscellaneous" for both Incident and Emergency Forms.

Exhibit 6-12. Incident Form – miscellaneous

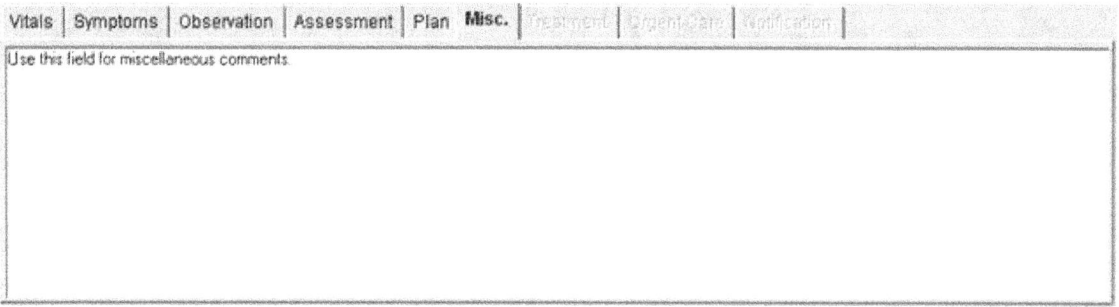

6.1.1 Incident Report Hard-Copy Form

Exhibit 6-13 is a hard-copy printout of an Incident Report Form.

Exhibit 6-13. Incident Report hard-copy form

Incident Report for Bobby Simone		02/14/1999

General Information

Person Type: SP	Recorder Name: Trumbore, Steve
Emergency Date: 02/14/1999	Runner Name(s):
Start Time: 10:25 AM End Time: 10:50 AM	Who Called 911:
Location: phlebotomy	Who Found: Edwards, Philessia
Description: fainted after blood draw	

Personal Info

Person ID: 589231	Age: 39	Gender: Male
Last name: Simone	First name: Bobby	Middle name:

Symptoms

Describe symptoms in this field

Vitals

Time:	Heart Rate:	Systolic:	Diastolic:	Respiratory Rate:	Comments:
10:30 AM	80	102	78	10	conscious, orientated x3, no injuries
10:40 AM	76	106	76	10	alert, orientated, wants to continue with exams

Observations

Describe observation in this field

Assessment

Describe assessment in this field.

Plan

Describe plan in this field

Miscellaneose

Use this field for miscellaneous comments.

6.2 Emergency Forms

The data entry for the Emergency Form (Exhibit 6-14) is similar to data entry for the Incident Form.

■ Select "Incident" or "Emergency" as appropriate.

■ Select the "Person Type." The choices are "SP," "Staff," or "Other." "Other" may include visitors or guests.

Exhibit 6-14. Emergency Form – blank

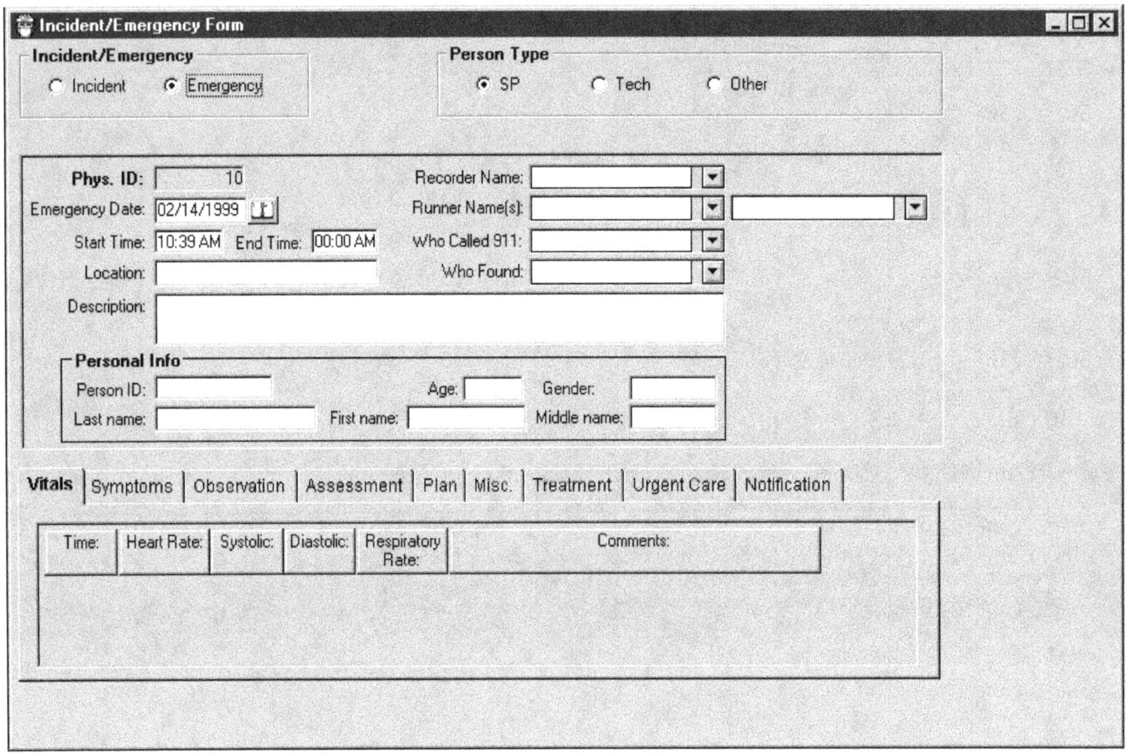

The "Date" is automatically entered as the current date. If the incident occurred earlier, the date entered should be the date the incident occurred. The date is a required field.

The "Start Time" is automatically entered as the time the form was opened. If the incident occurred earlier, the time entered should be the time the incident started. The "Start Time" is a required field. Please pay careful attention to this field in order to document the emergency accurately.

NOTE: "AM" is changed to "PM" by pressing "Shift-P" (press the Shift key and the P key) and "PM" is changed to "AM" by pressing "Shift A" (press the Shift key and the A key).

Exhibit 6-15 shows a completed Emergency Form. The "End Time" is the time the incident was resolved. This is a required field.

- Enter the location where the incident occurred in the "Location" field.

- Enter a brief description of the incident in the "Description" field.

- Enter the SP's (or staff) ID in the ID field and press the Tab key. The remainder of the "Personal Information" will be automatically entered.

- To add a line to enter "Vitals" information, right click (click the right button on the mouse) and select "Add" or "Insert." This may also be used to delete a line.

- Enter the time the vital signs were taken and then enter the heart rate/minute, systolic and diastolic blood pressure, and respiratory rate/minute.

- Enter a comment to describe the SP's condition at the time the vital signs were taken.

- Add more lines as necessary.

Exhibit 6-15. Emergency Form – data

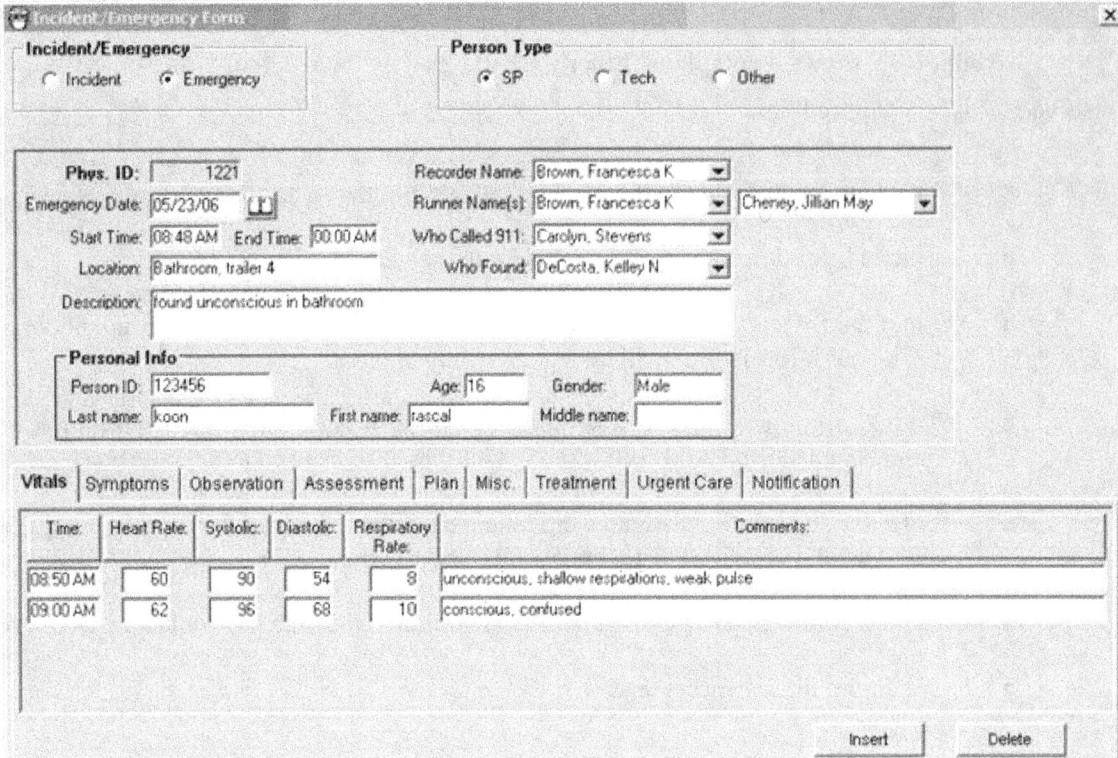

- Enter free text information in the Vitals, Symptoms, Observation, Assessment, Plan, and Miscellaneous fields.

- To add a line to enter "Treatment" information, right click (click the right button on the mouse) and select "Add" or "Insert." This may also be used to delete a line.

- Enter the time the treatment was administered.

- Select the "Medication" administered or "Equipment" used by clicking on the arrow to pull down the menu with the list of medications.

- Highlight the appropriate medication.

The medications in the emergency kit are displayed in Exhibits 6-16 and 6-17.

Exhibit 6-16. Emergency Report Form – treatment 1

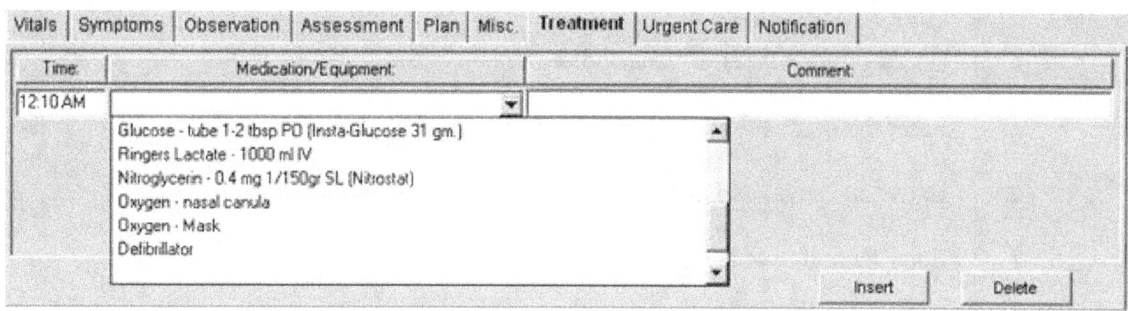

Exhibit 6-17. Emergency Report Form – treatment 2

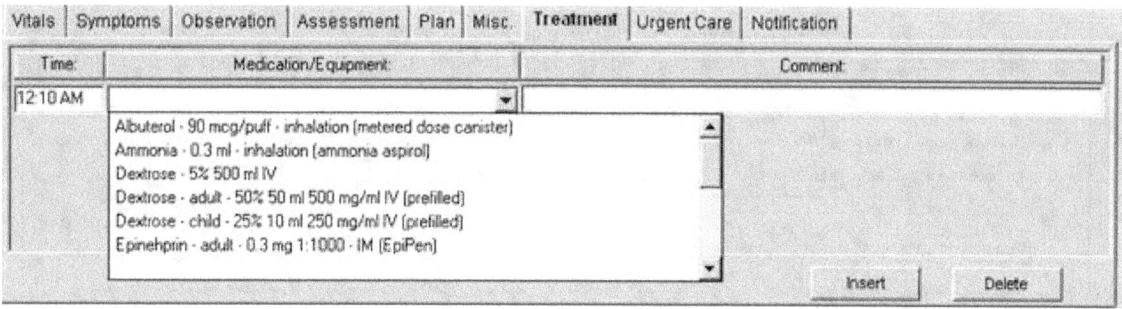

There are additional medications or equipment in the pick list for Emergency Medications/Equipment.

- If the SP needs to be transported to a hospital or clinic, click on the "Urgent Care" tab (Exhibit 6-18).

- Check the box labeled "Transported to hospital."

- Enter the name of the hospital in the "Hospital Name" field.

- Enter the arrival and departure time of the ambulance.

- Enter the name of the Emergency Service.

- Check the appropriate box if the physician accompanied the SP to the hospital.

Exhibit 6-18. Emergency Report Form – urgent care

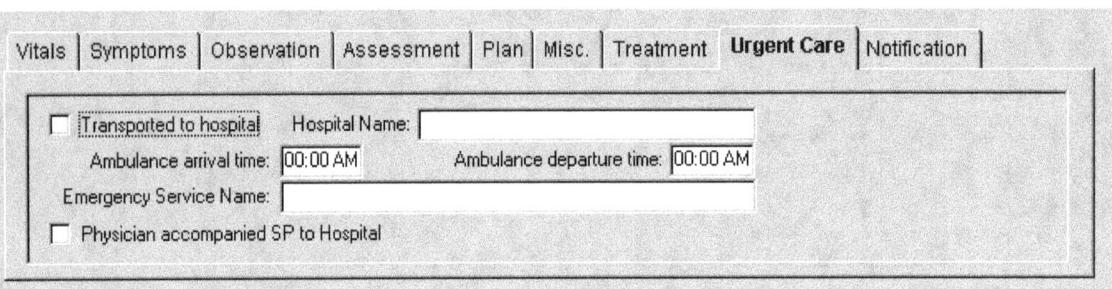

- Click on the "Notification" tab and enter information about notification of family member and/or physician (Exhibit 6-19).

Exhibit 6-19. Emergency Report Form – notification

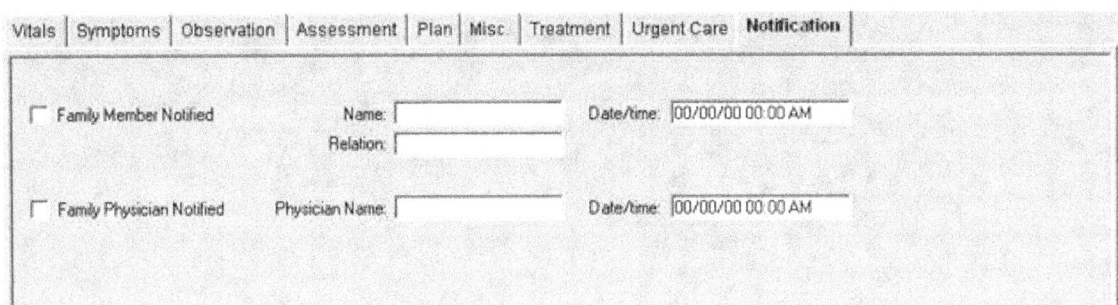

6.2.1 Emergency Report Hard-Copy Form

An example of the hard-copy printout (pages 1 and 2) of the Emergency Report Form is displayed in Exhibit 6-20.

Exhibit 6-20. Emergency Report hard-copy form

Emergency Report for Thomas Jefferson

02/14/1999

General Information

Person Type: SP

Emergency Date: 02/14/1999

Start Time: 10:44 AM   End Time: 11:30 AM

Location: Bathroom, trailer 4

Description: found unconscious in bathroom,

Recorder Name: Braddock, Ivy

Runner Name(s): Guerrero, Olga   Pinkerton, Ronald

Who Called 911: Trumbore, Steve

Who Found: Maples, Sean

Personal Info

Person ID: 705142

Last name: Jefferson

Age: 46

First name: Thomas

Gender: Male

Middle name:

Symptoms

Vitals

Time:	Heart Rate:	Systolic:	Diastolic:	Respiratory Rate:	Comments:
10:45 AM	52			8	unconscious, shallow respirations, weak pulse
10:50 AM	58	96	68	10	conscious , confused,

Observations

Describe observations in this field.

Assessment

Describe assessment in this field.

Plan

Describe plan in this field.

Miscellaneose

Additional field for miscellaneous comments.

Treatment

Time:	Medication/Equipment:	Comment:
10:45 AM	Oxygen - nasal canula	

Exhibit 6-20. Emergency Report hard-copy form (continued)

Emergency Report for Thomas Jefferson 02/14/1999

Urgent Care

☐ Transported to hospital   Hospital Name:

    Ambulance arrival time: 00:00 AM   Ambulance departure time: 00:00 AM

    Emergency service name:

☐ Physician accompanied SP to Hospital

Notification

☑ Family Member N   Name: Mary   Date/time: 02/14/99 11:00 AM

    Relation: wife

☑ Family Physician Notified

    Family Physican Name: Comstock   Date/time: 02/14/99 11:30 AM

7. QUALITY CONTROL

7.1   Elements of the Quality Control Program

To ensure complete and accurate data collection, the quality control program for this study will take place in mobile examination centers (MECs) and will consist of the following major elements:

- Training and calibrating of the physicians with gold standard expert;

- Monitoring equipment and equipment repair, and verifying weekly calibrations; and

- Site visit observations by NCHS and Westat.

7.2   Training and Calibrating of Physicians with Gold Standard Expert

The protocol for blood pressure measurement follows procedures developed by the American Heart Association. The physicians underwent initial training and certification in blood pressure measurement through a training program provided by an independent expert consultant. This certification process included didactic presentations, video presentations that included listening to and recording Korotkoff sounds, and practice listening to blood pressures of volunteers with a certified instructor. Certification is achieved when all requirements of the training program are met, as well as quarterly monitoring by the consultant. Ongoing training needs as identified by the home office staff and NCHS will be assessed and scheduled.

7.3   Monitoring Equipment and Equipment Repair

The equipment and room supplies need to be checked on a regular basis. Some checks are completed daily and others need only be completed weekly or at the beginning and end of each stand. These checks include calibration checks, maintenance inspection of equipment and supplies, and preparation of the room and equipment for the session exams. The specific timeframes for equipment QC are as follows: start of stand, daily, weekly, and end of stand.

All of the Quality Control (QC) processes are recorded in the computer application, which reminds the physicians to perform the time-sensitive QC procedures. If the QC procedures have not been completed for that period, this message will be displayed at each logon until the QC procedures have been completed for that time period. The home office component staff monitors the equipment QC completion rates and provides feedback and/or retraining as warranted.

Each time you log onto the application, the system will remind you to do Quality Control (QC) checks if the checks have not been completed for that time period. The specified QC checks performed at the beginning of stand, daily, weekly, and end of stand are selected by the physician. If you do not have time to do the checks when you logon, you can bypass this message and complete the checks at a later time. However, this message will be displayed each time you logon until you have completed the checks for that period. After you have completed the checks and entered this in the system, the message box with the remainder will not be displayed again until the appropriate time has passed.

7.3.1   Maintenance of Equipment

Physicians maintain all equipment used in their component. The following sections specifically state the requirements that physicians follow to check and maintain equipment used for the BP measurements. The following items are checked on a routine basis.

7.3.2   Inflation System (BP cuffs)

1.   Cuff material is clean, intact.

2.   Clean all cuffs with a disinfectant wipe.

3.   Velcro is functional and free of lint/debris.

4.   Rubber tubing and inflation bulb is smooth, has no cracks or tears.

5.   Pressure control valve opens and closes smoothly without sticking.

7.3.3   Littmann Cardiology III Stethoscopes

1.   Check the stethoscope for cracks in the tubing.

2.   Earpieces are securely attached.

3.   Head of stethoscope is securely attached to tubing.

4.   Diaphragm is secure, no cracks.

7.3.4   Mercury Sphygmomanometer

1. The shape of the meniscus (top of the column of mercury) should be a smooth, well-defined curve. If not, replace the equipment. This is usually caused by dirt/oxidation in the mercury or the glass tube.

2. Check that the mercury rises easily in the tubing and does not bounce noticeably when inflated. If the mercury does not rise easily in the tube, or if the column bounces noticeably as the valve is closed, replace the equipment.

3. Disconnect the inflation system from the cuff and confirm that the meniscus of the mercury in the glass manometer tube is zero.

4. Check for cracks in the glass tube.

5. Check the screw at the top of the calibrated glass tube to make sure it is securely in place.

6. Check the coiled air tube for cracks, tears.

7. Inflation system testing protocol to test for air leaks (test all BP cuffs in this manner):

   - Connect each size cuff to the inflation system and wrap it around the corresponding calibration cylinder;

   - Inflate to 250 mm Hg;

   - Open valve and deflate to 200 mm Hg and close valve;

   - Wait for 10 seconds; if mercury column drops more than 10 mm Hg, there is an air leak in the system; and

   - If a leak is detected, change the cuff, check the coiled tubing and repeat the test.

7.4   Frequency of QC Procedures

The designated intervals for the BP QC procedures are: start of stand, daily checks, weekly checks, and end of stand checks.

7.4.1 Daily QC Checks

1. Check to see if the level of mercury in glass tube is zero.

2. Check the shape of the meniscus.

3. Check that the mercury rises easily in the tubing and does not bounce noticeably.

4. Check for cracks in the glass tube.

5. Check that the cap at the top of the calibrated glass tube is secure.

6. Check pressure control valve for sticks or leaks.

7. Wipe both sides of BP cuffs with disinfectant wipes.

7.4.2 Weekly QC Checks

1. Complete daily checks.

2. Check functioning of all emergency equipment.

3. Complete inventory of emergency medications.

4. Check the cuffs, pressure bulb, and manometer and stethoscope tubing for cracks or tears.

5. Check stethoscope diaphragm for cracks.

6. Inflation system testing protocol to test for air leaks with the mercury manometer.

7.4.3 Start of Stand Checks

1. Complete daily checks.

2. Complete weekly checks.

7.4.4   End of Stand Checks

7.5   ISIS Data Entry Screens for QC on Equipment

7.5.1   Data Entry Screens for QC on Equipment

When you log onto the application (Exhibit 7-1) before the Quality Control checks are performed, the system displays a message: "One or more of your QC checks have not been performed."

Exhibit 7-1. Quality control logon with reminder message

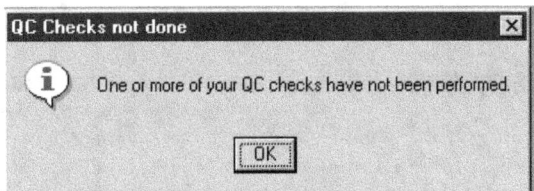

Click "OK" to this message. When you want to complete the QC checks, select "Utilities," then select Quality Control from the menu (Exhibit 7-2). Clicking on the QC icon from the Toolbar can also access the QC screens. When QC is selected from the Utilities menu, the Session Pick-Up box will be displayed. Select the current session.

Exhibit 7-2. Session Pick-Up Box

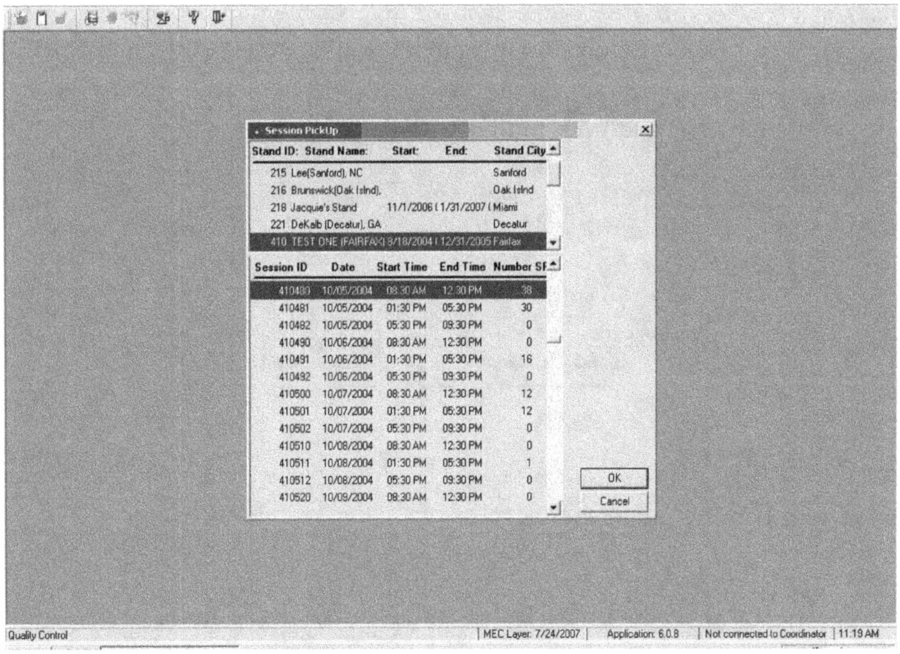

Each physician will have a personal ID. This ID will be used to identify the person who completed the QC checks for this time period. Enter your User ID and click "OK." If you do not want to do the QC checks at this time, click "Cancel." You will still be able to conduct the exam.

When you want to complete the QC checks, select "Utilities," then select Quality Control from the menu (Exhibit 7-3).

Clicking on the QC icon from the Toolbar can also access the QC screens.

Exhibit 7-3. Utilities menu to select Quality Control

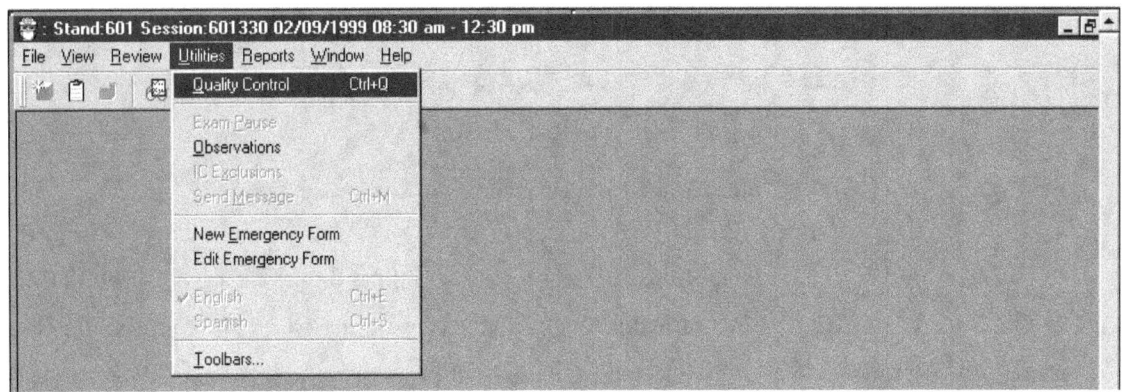

When QC is selected from the Utilities menu, the User ID entry box (Exhibit 7-4) will be displayed.

Exhibit 7-4. Quality Control log-on

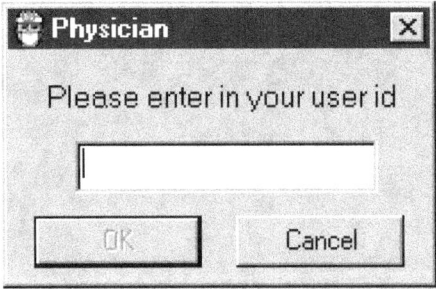

Enter your User ID and click "OK."

If you do not want to do the QC checks at this time, click "Cancel."

On the QC screens, check "Done" for the listed items when that item has been completed (Exhibit 7-5).

Exhibit 7-5. Example of a Quality Control screen

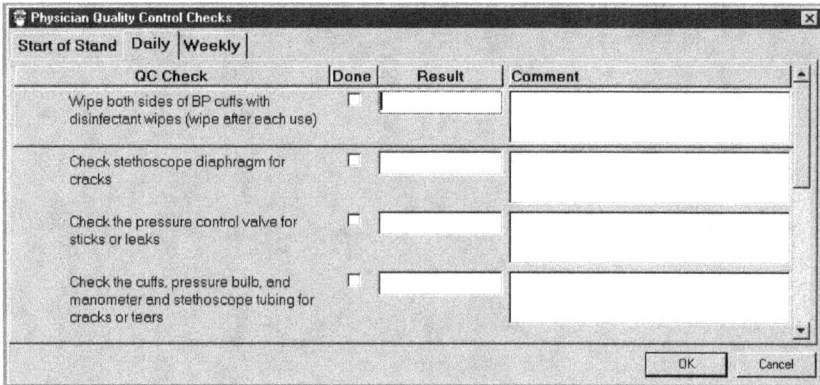

You are not required to enter anything in the "Result" or "Comment" fields unless there is a problem with the equipment. The "Result" field is used to enter values for selected QC items if required. The "Comments" field is used to enter information about problems encountered with the QC item check.

7.5.2   Daily Checks

On the QC daily checks screens, check "Done" for the listed items when that item has been completed (Exhibits 7-6 to 7-9).

Exhibit 7-6. Quality Control daily checks (1)

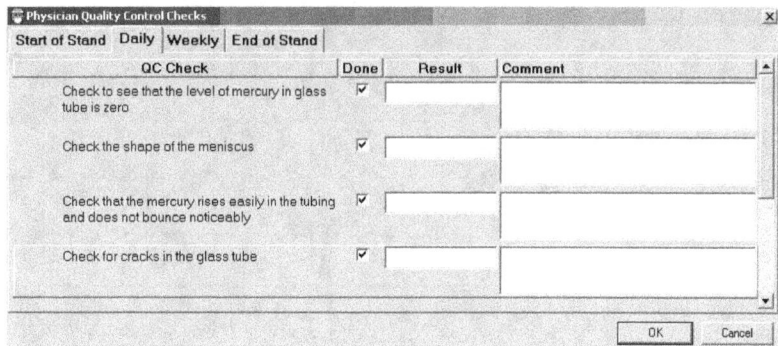

Exhibit 7-7. Quality Control daily checks (2)

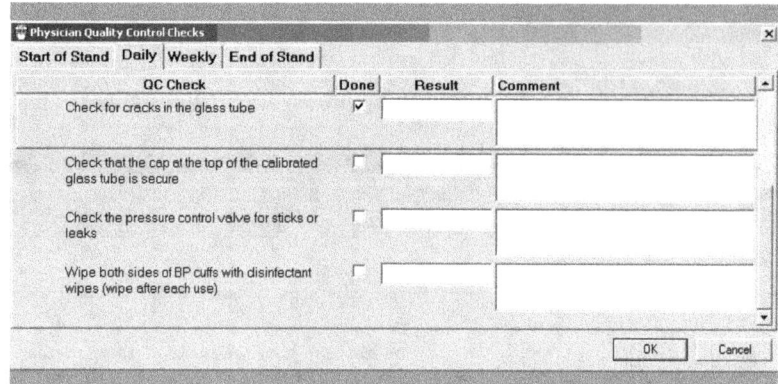

Use the scroll bar to move to the next item on the list.

Exhibit 7-8. Quality Control daily checks (3)

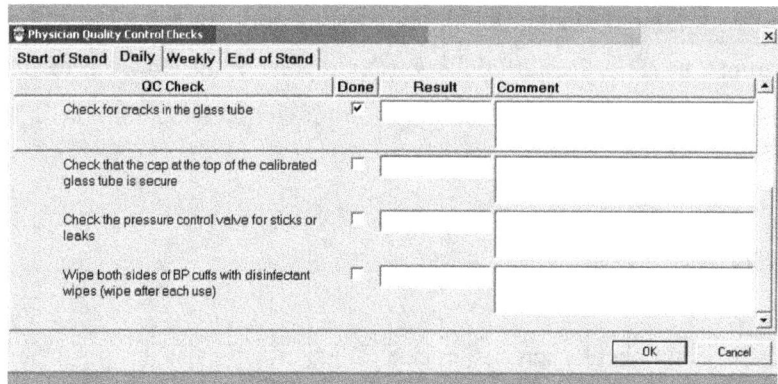

Exhibit 7-9. Quality Control daily checks (4)

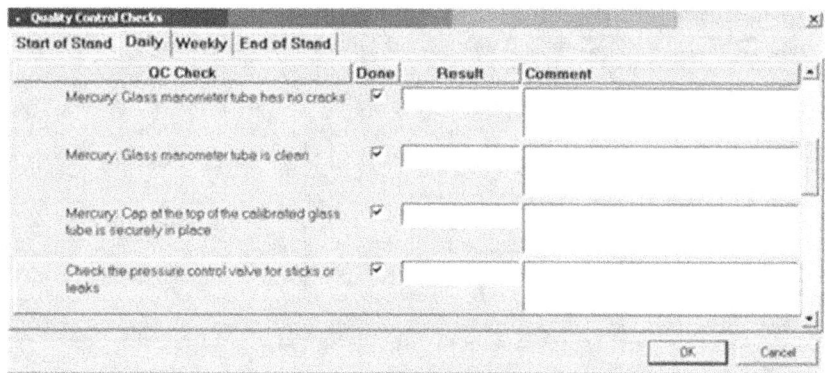

When you are finished with the daily item checks, click "OK" to close the QC box.

7.5.3 Weekly Checks

Use the scroll bar to move to the remaining items. When you are finished with the weekly item checks, click "OK" to close the QC box (Exhibit 7-10).

Exhibit 7-10. Quality Control weekly checks

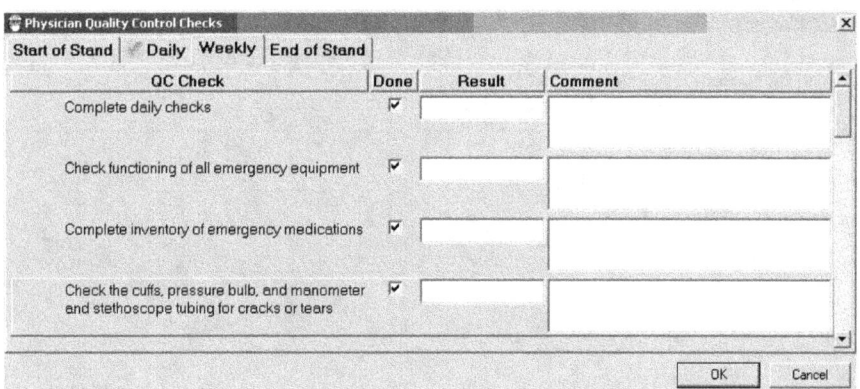

7.5.4 Start of Stand Checks

The start of stand checks are shown in Exhibit 7-11.

Exhibit 7-11. Quality Control start of stand checks

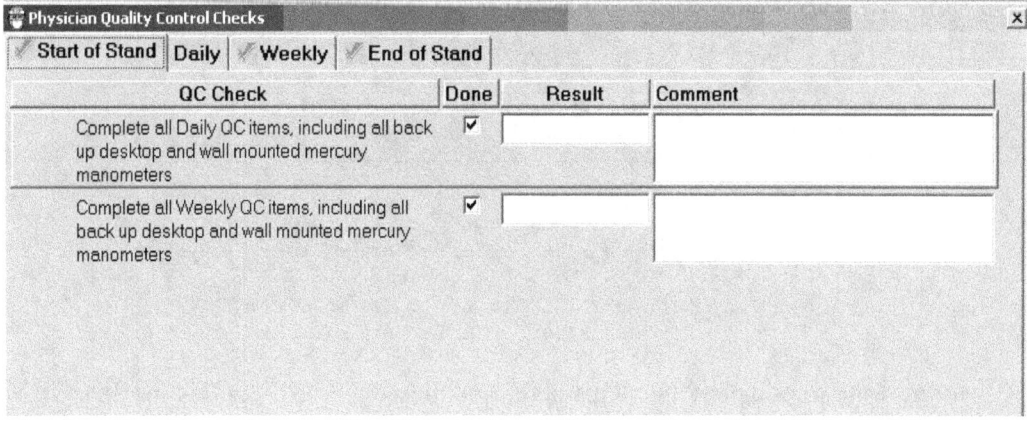

7.5.5   End of Stand Checks

The end of stand checks consist of the calibration screen in Exhibit 7-12.

Exhibit 7-12. Quality Control end of stand checks

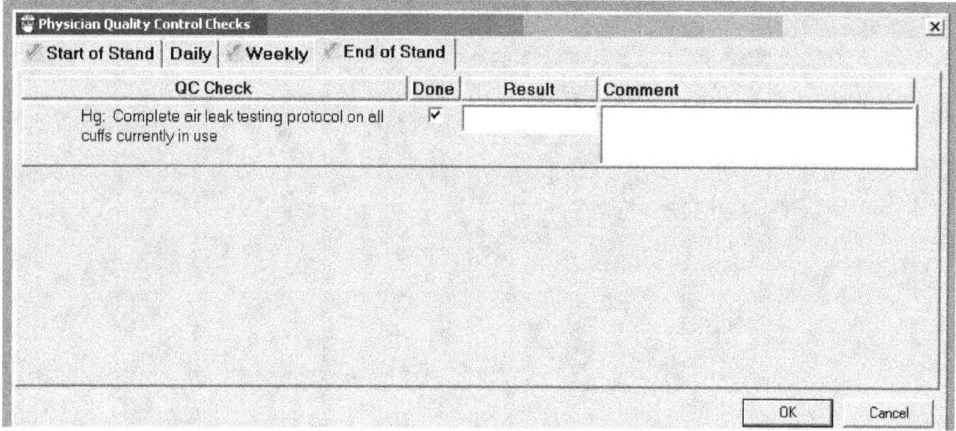

When you have completed all checks, click "OK" to close the QC box. If you do not check that all items are complete, the system will display this message: "Not all the QC items were done. Do you wish to exit?" (See Exhibit 7-13.)

Exhibit 7-13. Quality Control incomplete entry

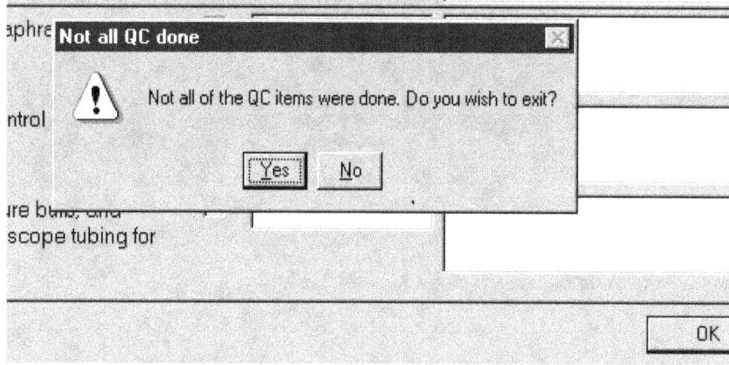

If you want to complete the items before exiting, click "No" to this message and complete the items. If you do not wish to complete all QC checks, click "Yes" to this message. If all QC items were not complete, the system will remind you each time you logon that the QC checks are not complete.

Below is a summary of the physician QC procedures.

Daily Checks:

1. Disconnect the inflation system from the cuff and confirm that the meniscus of the mercury in the glass manometer tube is zero;

2. Confirm that the shape of the mercury meniscus is a smooth, well-defined curve.

3. Check that the mercury rises easily in the tubing and mercury does not bounce noticeably when inflated.

4. Check for cracks in the glass tube.

5. Check the screw at the top of the calibrated glass tube to make sure it is securely in place.

6. Clean the cuffs with Sani-wipe cloths.

Weekly checks:

1. Complete daily checks.

2. Check functioning of emergency equipment: oxygen cylinders, AED.

3. Complete inventory of emergency medications:

Medication	Form supplied	Par Level
Albuterol (17g)	Metered dose canister	1
Ammonia	Ammonia Aspirol	1
Aspirin	Unit dose package	1
Diphenhydramine	Liquid	1
Diphenhydramine	Tablets	1
Epinephrine-adult	EpiPen	2
Epinephrine-peds	EpiPen Jr.	2
Glucose – tube	Insta-Glucose 31 gm	1
Nitroglycerin (25 tabs)	Nitrostat	1

4. Check Littmann Cardiology III Stethoscopes:

    -   Check the stethoscope for cracks in the tubing.

    -   Earpieces are securely attached.

    -   Head of stethoscope is securely attached to tubing.

    -   Diaphragm is secure, no cracks.

5. Check Inflation System & BP Cuffs:

    -   Cuff material is clean, intact.

    -   Velcro is functional and free of lint/debris.

    -   Rubber tubing and inflation bulb is smooth has no cracks or tears.

    -   Pressure control valve opens and closes smoothly without sticking.

    -   Check the coiled air tube for cracks, tears

6. Test mercury manometer and blood pressure cuffs for air leaks

    -   Wrap each size cuff around the corresponding calibration cylinder.

    -   Connect the cuffs to the manometer and inflate to 250 mm Hg.

    -   Check that the mercury rises easily in the tubing and does not bounce noticeably when inflated. If it does not rise easily in the tube, or if the mercury column bounces noticeably as the valve is closed, check connections, confirm that the pressure valve is closed, and re-test.

    -   Open valve and deflate to 200 mm Hg and close valve; and wait for 10 seconds; if mercury column drops more than 10 mm Hg, there is an air leak in the system.

    -   Repeat for each size cuff

    -   If a leak is detected, change the cuff, check the coiled tubing, check the inflation control valve on the cuff, confirm that all male/female connections are secure, and repeat the test.

Appendix A

Child Blood Pressure Values

APPENDIX A. CHILD BLOOD PRESSURE VALUES

Girls – Age 6

Percentile of height = Less than 10%

Systolic(mm Hg)	Diastolic (mm Hg)			
	<68	68 - 71	72 - 85	≥ 86
< 104	1	2	3	4
104 - 107	2	2	3	4
108 - 120	3	3	3	4
≥ 121	4	4	4	4

Percentile of height = 10 - 24%

Systolic(mm Hg)	Diastolic (mm Hg)			
	<68	68 - 71	72 - 85	≥ 86
< 105	1	2	3	4
105 - 108	2	2	3	4
109 - 121	3	3	3	4
≥ 122	4	4	4	4

Percentile of height = 25 - 49%

Systolic(mm Hg)	Diastolic (mm Hg)			
	<69	69 - 72	73 - 85	≥ 86
< 106	1	2	3	4
106 - 109	2	2	3	4
110 - 122	3	3	3	4
≥ 123	4	4	4	4

Percentile of height = 50 - 74%

Systolic(mm Hg)	Diastolic (mm Hg)			
	<70	70 - 73	74 - 86	≥ 87
< 108	1	2	3	4
108 - 110	2	2	3	4
111 - 124	3	3	3	4
≥ 125	4	4	4	4

Child Blood Pressure Values
Girls - Age 6 (continued)

Percentile of height = 75 - 89%

Systolic(mm Hg)	Diastolic (mm Hg)			
	<70	70 - 73	74 - 87	≥ 88
< 109	1	2	3	4
109 - 112	2	2	3	4
113 - 125	3	3	3	4
≥ 126	4	4	4	4

Percentile of height = 90 - 94%

Systolic(mm Hg)	Diastolic (mm Hg)			
	<71	71 - 74	75 - 88	≥ 89
< 110	1	2	3	4
110 - 113	2	2	3	4
114 - 126	3	3	3	4
≥ 127	4	4	4	4

Percentile of height = 95% and higher

Systolic(mm Hg)	Diastolic (mm Hg)			
	<72	72 - 75	76 - 88	≥ 89
< 111	1	2	3	4
111 - 114	2	2	3	4
115 - 127	3	3	3	4
≥ 128	4	4	4	4

Child Blood Pressure Values
Girls - Age 7

Percentile of height = Less than 10%

Systolic(mm Hg)	Diastolic (mm Hg)			
	<69	69 - 72	73 - 86	≥ 87
< 106	1	2	3	4
106 - 109	2	2	3	4
110 - 122	3	3	3	4
≥ 123	4	4	4	4

Percentile of height = 10 - 24%

Systolic(mm Hg)	Diastolic (mm Hg)			
	<70	70 - 73	74 - 86	≥ 87
< 107	1	2	3	4
107 - 110	2	2	3	4
111 - 123	3	3	3	4
≥ 124	4	4	4	4

Percentile of height = 25 - 49%

Systolic(mm Hg)	Diastolic (mm Hg)			
	<70	70 - 73	73 - 87	≥ 88
< 108	1	2	3	4
108 - 111	2	2	3	4
112 - 124	3	3	3	4
≥ 125	4	4	4	4

Percentile of height = 50 - 74%

Systolic(mm Hg)	Diastolic (mm Hg)			
	<71	71 - 74	75 - 87	≥ 88
< 109	1	2	3	4
109 - 112	2	2	3	4
113 - 125	3	3	3	4
≥ 126	4	4	4	4

Percentile of height = 75 - 89%

Systolic(mm Hg)	Diastolic (mm Hg)			
	<72	72 - 75	76 - 88	≥ 89
< 111	1	2	3	4
111 - 114	2	2	3	4
115 - 127	3	3	3	4
≥ 128	4	4	4	4

Percentile of height = 90 - 94%

Systolic(mm Hg)	Diastolic (mm Hg)			
	<72	72 - 75	76 - 89	≥ 90
< 112	1	2	3	4
112 - 115	2	2	3	4
116 - 128	3	3	3	4
≥ 129	4	4	4	4

Percentile of height = 95% and higher

Systolic(mm Hg)	Diastolic (mm Hg)			
	<73	73 - 76	77 - 89	≥ 90
< 113	1	2	3	4
113 - 115	2	2	3	4
116 - 129	3	3	3	4
≥ 130	4	4	4	4

Child Blood Pressure Values
Girls - Age 8

Percentile of height = Less than 10%

Systolic(mm Hg)	Diastolic (mm Hg)			
	<71	71 - 74	75 - 87	≥ 88
< 108	1	2	3	4
108 - 111	2	2	3	4
112 - 124	3	3	3	4
≥ 125	4	4	4	4

Percentile of height = 10 - 24%

Systolic(mm Hg)	Diastolic (mm Hg)			
	<71	71 - 74	75 - 87	≥ 88
< 109	1	2	3	4
109 - 111	2	2	3	4
112 - 125	3	3	3	4
≥ 126	4	4	4	4

Percentile of height = 25 - 49%

Systolic(mm Hg)	Diastolic (mm Hg)			
	<71	71 - 74	75 - 88	≥ 89
< 110	1	2	3	4
110 - 113	2	2	3	4
114 - 126	3	3	3	4
≥ 127	4	4	4	4

Percentile of height = 50 - 74%

Systolic(mm Hg)	Diastolic (mm Hg)			
	<72	72 - 75	76 - 88	≥ 89
< 111	1	2	3	4
111 - 114	2	2	3	4
115 - 127	3	3	3	4
≥ 128	4	4	4	4

Percentile of height = 75 - 89%

Systolic(mm Hg)	Diastolic (mm Hg)			
	<73	73 - 76	77 - 89	≥ 90
< 113	1	2	3	4
113 - 115	2	2	3	4
116 - 128	3	3	3	4
≥ 129	4	4	4	4

Percentile of height = 90 - 94%

Systolic(mm Hg)	Diastolic (mm Hg)			
	<74	74 - 77	78 - 90	≥ 91
< 114	1	2	3	4
114 - 117	2	2	3	4
118 - 130	3	3	3	4
≥ 131	4	4	4	4

Percentile of height = 95% and higher

Systolic(mm Hg)	Diastolic (mm Hg)			
	<74	74 - 77	78 - 91	≥ 92
< 114	1	2	3	4
114 - 117	2	2	3	4
118 - 130	3	3	3	4
≥ 131	4	4	4	4

Child Blood Pressure Values
Girls - Age 9

Percentile of height = Less than 10%

Systolic(mm Hg)	Diastolic (mm Hg)			
	<72	72 - 75	76 - 88	≥ 89
< 110	1	2	3	4
110 - 113	2	2	3	4
114 - 126	3	3	3	4
≥ 127	4	4	4	4

Percentile of height = 10 - 24%

Systolic(mm Hg)	Diastolic (mm Hg)			
	<72	72 - 75	76 - 88	<89
< 110	1	2	3	4
110 - 113	2	2	3	4
114 - 126	3	3	3	4
≥ 127	4	4	4	4

Percentile of height = 25 - 49%

Systolic(mm Hg)	Diastolic (mm Hg)			
	<72	72 - 75	76 - 89	≥ 90
< 112	1	2	3	4
112 - 114	2	2	3	4
115 - 128	3	3	3	4
≥ 129	4	4	4	4

Percentile of height = 50 - 74%

Systolic(mm Hg)	Diastolic (mm Hg)			
	<73	73 - 76	77 - 89	≥ 90
< 113	1	2	3	4
113 - 116	2	2	3	4
117 - 129	3	3	3	4
≥ 130	4	4	4	4

Child Blood Pressure Values
Girls - Age 9 (continued)

Percentile of height = 75 - 89%

Systolic(mm Hg)	Diastolic (mm Hg)			
	<74	74 - 77	78 - 90	≥ 91
< 114	1	2	3	4
114 - 117	2	2	3	4
118 - 130	3	3	3	4
≥ 131	4	4	4	4

Percentile of height = 90 - 94%

Systolic(mm Hg)	Diastolic (mm Hg)			
	<75	75 - 78	79 - 91	≥ 92
< 116	1	2	3	4
116 - 118	2	2	3	4
119 - 132	3	3	3	4
≥ 133	4	4	4	4

Percentile of height = 95% and higher

Systolic(mm Hg)	Diastolic (mm Hg)			
	<75	75 - 78	79 - 92	≥ 93
< 116	1	2	3	4
116 - 119	2	2	3	4
120 - 132	3	3	3	4
≥ 133	4	4	4	4

Child Blood Pressure Values
Girls - Age 10

Percentile of height = Less than 10%

Systolic(mm Hg)	Diastolic (mm Hg)			
	<73	73 - 76	77 - 89	≥90
< 112	1	2	3	4
112 - 115	2	2	3	4
116 - 128	3	3	3	4
≥ 129	4	4	4	4

Percentile of height = 10 - 24%

Systolic(mm Hg)	Diastolic (mm Hg)			
	<73	73 - 76	77 - 89	≥90
< 112	1	2	3	4
112 - 115	2	2	3	4
116 - 128	3	3	3	4
≥ 129	4	4	4	4

Percentile of height = 25 - 49%

Systolic(mm Hg)	Diastolic (mm Hg)			
	<73	73 - 76	77 - 90	≥91
< 114	1	2	3	4
114 - 116	2	2	3	4
117 - 130	3	3	3	4
≥ 131	4	4	4	4

Percentile of height = 50 - 74%

Systolic(mm Hg)	Diastolic (mm Hg)			
	<74	74 - 77	78 - 91	≥ 92
< 115	1	2	3	4
115 - 118	2	2	3	4
119 - 131	3	3	3	4
≥ 132	4	4	4	4

Child Blood Pressure Values
Girls - Age 10 (continued)

Percentile of height = 75 - 89%

Systolic(mm Hg)	Diastolic (mm Hg)			
	<75	75 - 78	79 - 91	≥ 92
< 116	1	2	3	4
116 - 119	2	2	3	4
120 - 132	3	3	3	4
≥ 133	4	4	4	4

Percentile of height = 90 - 94%

Systolic(mm Hg)	Diastolic (mm Hg)			
	<76	76 - 79	80 - 92	≥ 93
< 118	1	2	3	4
118 - 120	2	2	3	4
121 - 134	3	3	3	4
≥ 135	4	4	4	4

Percentile of height = 95% and higher

Systolic(mm Hg)	Diastolic (mm Hg)			
	<76	76 - 79	80 - 93	≥ 94
< 118	1	2	3	4
118 - 121	2	2	3	4
122 - 134	3	3	3	4
≥ 135	4	4	4	4

Child Blood Pressure Values
Girls - Age 11

Percentile of height = Less than 10%

Systolic(mm Hg)	Diastolic (mm Hg)			
	<74	74 - 77	78 - 90	≥ 91
< 114	1	2	3	4
114 - 117	2	2	3	4
118 - 130	3	3	3	4
≥ 131	4	4	4	4

Percentile of height = 10 - 24%

Systolic(mm Hg)	Diastolic (mm Hg)			
	<74	74 - 77	78 - 90	≥ 91
< 114	1	2	3	4
114 - 117	2	2	3	4
118 - 130	3	3	3	4
≥ 131	4	4	4	4

Percentile of height = 25 - 49%

Systolic(mm Hg)	Diastolic (mm Hg)			
	<74	74 - 77	78 - 91	≥ 92
< 116	1	2	3	4
116 - 118	2	2	3	4
119 - 131	3	3	3	4
≥ 132	4	4	4	4

Percentile of height = 50 - 74%

Systolic(mm Hg)	Diastolic (mm Hg)			
	<75	75 - 78	79 - 92	≥ 93
< 117	1	2	3	4
117 - 120	2	2	3	4
121 - 133	3	3	3	4
≥ 134	4	4	4	4

Child Blood Pressure Values
Girls - Age 11 (continued)

Percentile of height = 75 - 89%

Systolic(mm Hg)	Diastolic (mm Hg)			
	<76	76 - 79	80 - 92	≥ 93
< 118	1	2	3	4
118 - 121	2	2	3	4
122 - 134	3	3	3	4
≥ 135	4	4	4	4

Percentile of height = 90 - 94%

Systolic(mm Hg)	Diastolic (mm Hg)			
	<77	77 - 80	81 - 93	≥ 94
< 119	1	2	3	4
119 - 122	2	2	3	4
123 - 135	3	3	3	4
≥ 136	4	4	4	4

Percentile of height = 95% and higher

Systolic(mm Hg)	Diastolic (mm Hg)			
	<77	77 - 80	81 - 94	≥ 95
< 120	1	2	3	4
120 - 123	2	2	3	4
124 - 136	3	3	3	4
≥ 137	4	4	4	4

Child Blood Pressure Values
Girls - Age 12

Percentile of height = Less than 10%

Systolic(mm Hg)	Diastolic (mm Hg)			
	<75	75 - 78	79 - 91	≥ 92
< 116	1	2	3	4
116 - 118	2	2	3	4
119 - 132	3	3	3	4
≥ 133	4	4	4	4

Percentile of height = 10 - 24%

Systolic(mm Hg)	Diastolic (mm Hg)			
	<75	75 - 78	79 - 91	≥ 92
< 116	1	2	3	4
116 - 119	2	2	3	4
120 - 132	3	3	3	4
≥ 133	4	4	4	4

Percentile of height = 25 - 49%

Systolic(mm Hg)	Diastolic (mm Hg)			
	<75	75 - 78	79 - 92	≥ 93
< 117	1	2	3	4
117 - 120	2	2	3	4
121 - 133	3	3	3	4
≥ 134	4	4	4	4

Percentile of height = 50 - 74%

Systolic(mm Hg)	Diastolic (mm Hg)			
	<76	76 - 79	80 - 93	≥94
< 119	1	2	3	4
119 - 122	2	2	3	4
123 - 135	3	3	3	4
≥ 136	4	4	4	4

Child Blood Pressure Values
Girls - Age 12 (continued)

Percentile of height = 75 - 89%

Systolic(mm Hg)	Diastolic (mm Hg)			
	<77	77 - 80	81 - 93	≥ 94
< 120	1	2	3	4
120 - 123	2	2	3	4
124 - 136	3	3	3	4
≥ 137	4	4	4	4

Percentile of height = 90 - 94%

Systolic(mm Hg)	Diastolic (mm Hg)			
	<78	78 - 81	82 - 94	≥ 95
< 120	1	2	3	4
120 - 124	2	2	3	4
125 - 137	3	3	3	4
≥ 138	4	4	4	4

Percentile of height = 95% and higher

Systolic(mm Hg)	Diastolic (mm Hg)			
	<78	78 - 81	82 - 95	≥ 96
< 120	1	2	3	4
120 - 125	2	2	3	4
126 - 138	3	3	3	4
≥ 139	4	4	4	4

Child Blood Pressure Values
Girls - Age 13

Percentile of height = Less than 10%

Systolic(mm Hg)	Diastolic (mm Hg)			
	<76	76 - 79	80 - 92	≥ 93
< 117	1	2	3	4
117 - 120	2	2	3	4
121 - 133	3	3	3	4
≥ 134	4	4	4	4

Percentile of height = 10 - 24%

Systolic(mm Hg)	Diastolic (mm Hg)			
	<76	76 - 79	80 - 92	≥ 93
< 118	1	2	3	4
118 - 121	2	2	3	4
122 - 134	3	3	3	4
≥ 135	4	4	4	4

Percentile of height = 25 - 49%

Systolic(mm Hg)	Diastolic (mm Hg)			
	<76	76 - 79	80 - 93	≥ 94
< 119	1	2	3	4
119 - 122	2	2	3	4
123 - 135	3	3	3	4
≥ 136	4	4	4	4

Percentile of height = 50 - 74%

Systolic(mm Hg)	Diastolic (mm Hg)			
	<77	77 - 80	81 - 94	≥ 95
< 120	1	2	3	4
120 - 123	2	2	3	4
124 - 137	3	3	3	4
≥ 138	4	4	4	4

Child Blood Pressure Values
Girls - Age 13 (continued)

Percentile of height = 75 - 89%

Systolic(mm Hg)	Diastolic (mm Hg)			
	<78	78 - 81	82 - 94	≥ 95
< 120	1	2	3	4
120 - 125	2	2	3	4
126 - 138	3	3	3	4
≥ 139	4	4	4	4

Percentile of height = 90 - 94%

Systolic(mm Hg)	Diastolic (mm Hg)			
	<79	79 - 82	83 - 95	≥ 96
< 120	1	2	3	4
120 - 126	2	2	3	4
127 - 139	3	3	3	4
≥ 140	4	4	4	4

Percentile of height = 95% and higher

Systolic(mm Hg)	Diastolic (mm Hg)			
	<79	79 - 82	83 - 96	≥ 97
< 120	1	2	3	4
120 - 127	2	2	3	4
128 - 140	3	3	3	4
≥ 141	4	4	4	4

Child Blood Pressure Values
Girls - Age 14

Percentile of height = Less than 10%

Systolic(mm Hg)	Diastolic (mm Hg)			
	<77	77 - 80	81 - 93	≥ 94
< 119	1	2	3	4
119 - 122	2	2	3	4
123 - 135	3	3	3	4
≥ 136	4	4	4	4

Percentile of height = 10 - 24%

Systolic(mm Hg)	Diastolic (mm Hg)			
	<77	77 - 80	81 - 93	≥ 94
< 120	1	2	3	4
120 - 122	2	2	3	4
123 - 136	3	3	3	4
≥ 137	4	4	4	4

Percentile of height = 25 - 49%

Systolic(mm Hg)	Diastolic (mm Hg)			
	<77	77 - 80	81 - 94	≥ 95
< 120	1	2	3	4
120 - 124	2	2	3	4
125 - 137	3	3	3	4
≥ 138	4	4	4	4

Percentile of height = 50 - 74%

Systolic(mm Hg)	Diastolic (mm Hg)			
	<78	78 - 81	82 - 95	≥ 96
< 120	1	2	3	4
120 - 125	2	2	3	4
126 - 138	3	3	3	4
≥ 139	4	4	4	4

Child Blood Pressure Values
Girls - Age 14 (continued)

Percentile of height = 75 - 89%

Systolic(mm Hg)	Diastolic (mm Hg)			
	<79	79 - 82	83 - 95	≥ 96
< 120	1	2	3	4
120 - 126	2	2	3	4
127 - 140	3	3	3	4
≥ 141	4	4	4	4

Percentile of height = 90 - 94%

Systolic(mm Hg)	Diastolic (mm Hg)			
	<80	80 - 83	84 - 96	≥ 97
< 120	1	2	3	4
120 - 128	2	2	3	4
129 - 141	3	3	3	4
≥ 142	4	4	4	4

Percentile of height = 95% and higher

Systolic(mm Hg)	Diastolic (mm Hg)			
	<80	80 - 83	84 - 97	≥ 98
< 120	1	2	3	4
120 - 128	2	2	3	4
129 - 141	3	3	3	4
≥ 142	4	4	4	4

Child Blood Pressure Values
Girls - Age 15

Percentile of height = Less than 10%

Systolic(mm Hg)	Diastolic (mm Hg)			
	<78	78 - 81	82 - 94	≥ 95
< 120	1	2	3	4
120 - 123	2	2	3	4
124 - 136	3	3	3	4
≥ 137	4	4	4	4

Percentile of height = 10 - 24%

Systolic(mm Hg)	Diastolic (mm Hg)			
	<78	78 - 81	82 - 94	≥ 95
< 120	1	2	3	4
120 - 124	2	2	3	4
125 - 137	3	3	3	4
≥ 138	4	4	4	4

Percentile of height = 25 - 49%

Systolic(mm Hg)	Diastolic (mm Hg)			
	<78	78 - 81	82 - 95	≥ 96
< 120	1	2	3	4
120 - 125	2	2	3	4
126 - 138	3	3	3	4
≥ 139	4	4	4	4

Percentile of height = 50 - 74%

Systolic(mm Hg)	Diastolic (mm Hg)			
	<79	79 - 83	84 - 96	≥ 97
< 120	1	2	3	4
120 - 126	2	2	3	4
127 - 139	3	3	3	4
≥ 140	4	4	4	4

Child Blood Pressure Values
Girls - Age 15 (continued)

Percentile of height = 75 - 89%

Systolic(mm Hg)	Diastolic (mm Hg)			
	<80	80 - 84	85 - 97	≥ 98
< 120	1	2	3	4
120 - 128	2	2	3	4
129 - 141	3	3	3	4
≥ 142	4	4	4	4

Percentile of height = 90 - 94%

Systolic(mm Hg)	Diastolic (mm Hg)			
	<80	80 - 84	85 - 97	≥ 98
< 120	1	2	3	4
120 - 129	2	2	3	4
130 - 142	3	3	3	4
≥ 143	4	4	4	4

Percentile of height = 95% and higher

Systolic(mm Hg)	Diastolic (mm Hg)			
	<80	80 - 84	85 - 98	≥ 99
< 120	1	2	3	4
120 - 130	2	2	3	4
131 - 143	3	3	3	4
≥ 144	4	4	4	4

Child Blood Pressure Values
Girls - Age 16

Percentile of height = Less than 10%

Systolic(mm Hg)	Diastolic (mm Hg)			
	<78	78 - 81	82 - 95	≥ 96
< 120	1	2	3	4
120 - 124	2	2	3	4
125 - 137	3	3	3	4
≥ 138	4	4	4	4

Percentile of height = 10 - 24%

Systolic(mm Hg)	Diastolic (mm Hg)			
	<78	78 - 81	82 - 95	≥ 96
< 120	1	2	3	4
120 - 125	2	2	3	4
126 - 138	3	3	3	4
≥ 139	4	4	4	4

Percentile of height = 25 - 49%

Systolic(mm Hg)	Diastolic (mm Hg)			
	<79	79 - 82	83 - 95	≥ 96
< 120	1	2	3	4
120 - 126	2	2	3	4
127 - 139	3	3	3	4
≥ 140	4	4	4	4

Percentile of height = 50 - 74%

Systolic(mm Hg)	Diastolic (mm Hg)			
	<80	80 - 83	84 - 96	≥ 97
< 120	1	2	3	4
120 - 127	2	2	3	4
128 - 140	3	3	3	4
≥ 141	4	4	4	4

Child Blood Pressure Values
Girls - Age 16 (continued)

Percentile of height = 75 - 89%

Systolic(mm Hg)	Diastolic (mm Hg)			
	<80	80 - 84	85 - 97	≥ 98
< 120	1	2	3	4
120 - 129	2	2	3	4
130 - 142	3	3	3	4
≥ 143	4	4	4	4

Percentile of height = 90 - 94%

Systolic(mm Hg)	Diastolic (mm Hg)			
	<80	80 - 84	85 - 98	≥ 99
< 120	1	2	3	4
120 - 130	2	2	3	4
131 - 143	3	3	3	4
≥ 144	4	4	4	4

Percentile of height = 95% and higher

Systolic(mm Hg)	Diastolic (mm Hg)			
	<80	80 - 85	86 - 98	≥ 99
< 120	1	2	3	4
120 - 131	2	2	3	4
132 - 144	3	3	3	4
≥ 145	4	4	4	4

Child Blood Pressure Values
Girls - Age 17

Percentile of height = Less than 10%

Systolic(mm Hg)	Diastolic (mm Hg)			
	<78	78 - 81	82 - 95	≥ 96
< 120	1	2	3	4
120 - 124	2	2	3	4
125 - 138	3	3	3	4
≥ 139	4	4	4	4

Percentile of height = 10 - 24%

Systolic(mm Hg)	Diastolic (mm Hg)			
	<79	79 - 82	83 - 95	≥ 96
< 120	1	2	3	4
120 - 125	2	2	3	4
126 - 138	3	3	3	4
≥ 139	4	4	4	4

Percentile of height = 25 - 49%

Systolic(mm Hg)	Diastolic (mm Hg)			
	<79	79 - 82	83 - 96	≥ 97
< 120	1	2	3	4
120 - 126	2	2	3	4
127 - 139	3	3	3	4
≥ 140	4	4	4	4

Percentile of height = 50 - 74%

Systolic(mm Hg)	Diastolic (mm Hg)			
	<80	80 - 83	84 - 96	≥ 97
< 120	1	2	3	4
120 - 128	2	2	3	4
129 - 141	3	3	3	4
≥ 142	4	4	4	4

Child Blood Pressure Values
Girls - Age 17 (continued)

Percentile of height = 75 - 89%

Systolic(mm Hg)	Diastolic (mm Hg)			
	<80	80 - 84	85 - 97	≥ 98
< 120	1	2	3	4
120 - 129	2	2	3	4
130 - 142	3	3	3	4
≥ 143	4	4	4	4

Percentile of height = 90 - 94%

Systolic(mm Hg)	Diastolic (mm Hg)			
	<80	80 - 85	86 - 98	≥ 99
< 120	1	2	3	4
120 - 130	2	2	3	4
131 - 143	3	3	3	4
≥ 144	4	4	4	4

Percentile of height = 95% and higher

Systolic(mm Hg)	Diastolic (mm Hg)			
	<80	80 - 85	86 - 98	≥ 99
< 120	1	2	3	4
120 - 131	2	2	3	4
132 - 144	3	3	3	4
≥ 145	4	4	4	4

Child Blood Pressure Values
Boys - Age 6

Percentile of height = Less than 10%

Systolic(mm Hg)	Diastolic (mm Hg)			
	<68	68 - 71	72 - 85	≥ 86
< 105	1	2	3	4
105 - 108	2	2	3	4
109 - 121	3	3	3	4
≥ 122	4	4	4	4

Percentile of height = 10 - 24%

Systolic(mm Hg)	Diastolic (mm Hg)			
	<68	68 - 71	72 - 85	≥ 86
< 106	1	2	3	4
106 - 109	2	2	3	4
110 - 122	3	3	3	4
≥ 123	4	4	4	4

Percentile of height = 25 - 49%

Systolic(mm Hg)	Diastolic (mm Hg)			
	<69	69 - 72	73 - 86	≥ 87
< 108	1	2	3	4
108 - 111	2	2	3	4
112 - 124	3	3	3	4
≥ 125	4	4	4	4

Percentile of height = 50 - 74%

Systolic(mm Hg)	Diastolic (mm Hg)			
	<70	70 - 73	74 - 87	≥ 88
< 110	1	2	3	4
110 - 113	2	2	3	4
114 - 126	3	3	3	4
≥ 127	4	4	4	4

Child Blood Pressure Values
Boys - Age 6 (continued)

Percentile of height = 75 - 89%

Systolic(mm Hg)	Diastolic (mm Hg)			
	<71	71 - 74	75 - 88	≥ 89
< 111	1	2	3	4
111 - 114	2	2	3	4
115 - 128	3	3	3	4
≥ 129	4	4	4	4

Percentile of height = 90 - 94%

Systolic(mm Hg)	Diastolic (mm Hg)			
	<72	72 - 75	76 - 90	≥ 91
< 113	1	2	3	4
113 - 116	2	2	3	4
117 - 129	3	3	3	4
≥ 130	4	4	4	4

Percentile of height = 95% and higher

Systolic(mm Hg)	Diastolic (mm Hg)			
	<72	72 - 75	76 - 89	≥ 90
< 113	1	2	3	4
113 - 116	2	2	3	4
117 - 130	3	3	3	4
≥ 131	4	4	4	4

Child Blood Pressure Values
Boys - Age 7

Percentile of height = Less than 10%

Systolic(mm Hg)	Diastolic (mm Hg)			
	<70	70 - 73	74 - 87	≥ 88
< 106	1	2	3	4
106 - 109	2	2	3	4
110 - 122	3	3	3	4
≥ 123	4	4	4	4

Percentile of height = 10 - 24%

Systolic(mm Hg)	Diastolic (mm Hg)			
	<70	70 - 73	74 - 87	<88
< 107	1	2	3	4
107 - 110	2	2	3	4
111 - 121	3	3	3	4
≥ 122	4	4	4	4

Percentile of height = 25 - 49%

Systolic(mm Hg)	Diastolic (mm Hg)			
	<71	71 - 74	75 - 88	≥ 89
< 109	1	2	3	4
109 - 112	2	2	3	4
113 - 125	3	3	3	4
≥ 126	4	4	4	4

Percentile of height = 50 - 74%

Systolic(mm Hg)	Diastolic (mm Hg)			
	<72	72 - 75	76 - 89	≥ 90
< 111	1	2	3	4
111 - 114	2	2	3	4
115 - 127	3	3	3	4
≥ 128	4	4	4	4

Child Blood Pressure Values
Boys - Age 7 (continued)

Percentile of height = 75 - 89%

Systolic(mm Hg)	Diastolic (mm Hg)			
	<73	73 - 76	77 - 90	≥ 91
< 113	1	2	3	4
113 - 116	2	2	3	4
117 - 129	3	3	3	4
≥ 130	4	4	4	4

Percentile of height = 90 - 94%

Systolic(mm Hg)	Diastolic (mm Hg)			
	<74	74 - 77	78 - 91	≥ 92
< 114	1	2	3	4
114 - 117	2	2	3	4
118 - 130	3	3	3	4
≥ 131	4	4	4	4

Percentile of height = 95% and higher

Systolic(mm Hg)	Diastolic (mm Hg)			
	<74	74 - 77	78 - 91	≥ 92
< 115	1	2	3	4
115 - 118	2	2	3	4
119 - 131	3	3	3	4
≥ 132	4	4	4	4

Child Blood Pressure Values
Boys - Age 8

Percentile of height = Less than 10%

Systolic(mm Hg)	Diastolic (mm Hg)			
	<71	71 - 74	75 - 88	≥ 89
< 107	1	2	3	4
107 - 110	2	2	3	4
111 - 124	3	3	3	4
≥ 125	4	4	4	4

Percentile of height = 10 - 24%

Systolic(mm Hg)	Diastolic (mm Hg)			
	<72	72 - 75	76 - 89	≥ 90
< 109	1	2	3	4
109 - 111	2	2	3	4
112 - 125	3	3	3	4
≥ 126	4	4	4	4

Percentile of height = 25 - 49%

Systolic(mm Hg)	Diastolic (mm Hg)			
	<72	72 - 76	77 - 90	≥ 91
< 110	1	2	3	4
110 - 113	2	2	3	4
114 - 127	3	3	3	4
≥ 128	4	4	4	4

Percentile of height = 50 - 74%

Systolic(mm Hg)	Diastolic (mm Hg)			
	<73	73 - 77	78 - 91	≥ 92
< 112	1	2	3	4
112 - 115	2	2	3	4
116 - 128	3	3	3	4
≥ 129	4	4	4	4

Percentile of height = 75 - 89%

Systolic(mm Hg)	Diastolic (mm Hg)			
	<74	74 - 78	79 - 92	≥ 93
< 114	1	2	3	4
114 - 117	2	2	3	4
118 - 130	3	3	3	4
≥ 131	4	4	4	4

Percentile of height = 90 - 94%

Systolic(mm Hg)	Diastolic (mm Hg)			
	<75	75 - 78	79 - 92	≥ 93
< 115	1	2	3	4
115 - 118	2	2	3	4
119 - 132	3	3	3	4
≥ 133	4	4	4	4

Percentile of height = 95% and higher

Systolic(mm Hg)	Diastolic (mm Hg)			
	<76	76 - 79	80 - 93	≥ 94
< 116	1	2	3	4
116 - 119	2	2	3	4
120 - 132	3	3	3	4
≥ 133	4	4	4	4

Child Blood Pressure Values
Boys - Age 9

Percentile of height = Less than 10%

Systolic(mm Hg)	Diastolic (mm Hg)			
	<72	72 - 75	76 - 89	≥ 90
< 109	1	2	3	4
109 - 112	2	2	3	4
113 - 125	3	3	3	4
≥ 126	4	4	4	4

Percentile of height = 10 - 24%

Systolic(mm Hg)	Diastolic (mm Hg)			
	<73	73 - 76	77 - 90	<91
< 110	1	2	3	4
110 - 113	2	2	3	4
114 - 126	3	3	3	4
≥ 127	4	4	4	4

Percentile of height = 25 - 49%

Systolic(mm Hg)	Diastolic (mm Hg)			
	<74	74 - 77	78 - 91	≥ 92
< 112	1	2	3	4
112 - 115	2	2	3	4
116 - 128	3	3	3	4
≥ 129	4	4	4	4

Percentile of height = 50 - 74%

Systolic(mm Hg)	Diastolic (mm Hg)			
	<75	75 - 78	79 - 92	≥ 93
< 114	1	2	3	4
114 - 117	2	2	3	4
118 - 130	3	3	3	4
≥ 131	4	4	4	4

Child Blood Pressure Values
Boys - Age 9 (continued)

Percentile of height = 75 - 89%

Systolic(mm Hg)	Diastolic (mm Hg)			
	<75	75 - 79	80 - 86	≥ 87
< 115	1	2	3	4
115 - 118	2	2	3	4
119 - 132	3	3	3	4
≥ 133	4	4	4	4

Percentile of height = 90 - 94%

Systolic(mm Hg)	Diastolic (mm Hg)			
	<76	76 - 79	80 - 93	≥ 94
< 117	1	2	3	4
117 - 120	2	2	3	4
121 - 133	3	3	3	4
≥ 134	4	4	4	4

Percentile of height = 95% and higher

Systolic(mm Hg)	Diastolic (mm Hg)			
	<77	77 - 80	81 - 94	≥ 95
< 118	1	2	3	4
118 - 120	2	2	3	4
121 - 134	3	3	3	4
≥ 135	4	4	4	4

Child Blood Pressure Values
Boys - Age 10

Percentile of height = Less than 10%

Systolic(mm Hg)	Diastolic (mm Hg)			
	<73	73 - 76	77 - 90	≥ 91
< 111	1	2	3	4
111 - 114	2	2	3	4
115 - 127	3	3	3	4
≥ 128	4	4	4	4

Percentile of height = 10 - 24%

Systolic(mm Hg)	Diastolic (mm Hg)			
	<73	73 - 77	78 - 91	≥ 92
< 112	1	2	3	4
112 - 115	2	2	3	4
116 - 128	3	3	3	4
≥ 129	4	4	4	4

Percentile of height = 25 - 49%

Systolic(mm Hg)	Diastolic (mm Hg)			
	<74	74 - 78	79 - 91	≥ 92
< 114	1	2	3	4
114 - 116	2	2	3	4
117 - 130	3	3	3	4
≥ 131	4	4	4	4

Percentile of height = 50 - 74%

Systolic(mm Hg)	Diastolic (mm Hg)			
	<75	75 - 79	80 - 93	≥ 94
< 115	1	2	3	4
115 - 118	2	2	3	4
119 - 132	3	3	3	4
≥ 133	4	4	4	4

Child Blood Pressure Values
Boys - Age 10 (continued)

Percentile of height = 75 - 89%

Systolic(mm Hg)	Diastolic (mm Hg)			
	<76	76 - 80	81 - 93	≥ 94
< 117	1	2	3	4
117 - 120	2	2	3	4
121 - 133	3	3	3	4
≥ 134	4	4	4	4

Percentile of height = 90 - 94%

Systolic(mm Hg)	Diastolic (mm Hg)			
	<77	77 - 80	81 - 94	≥ 95
< 119	1	2	3	4
119 - 121	2	2	3	4
122 - 135	3	3	3	4
≥ 136	4	4	4	4

Percentile of height = 95% and higher

Systolic(mm Hg)	Diastolic (mm Hg)			
	<78	78 - 81	82 - 95	≥ 96
< 119	1	2	3	4
119 - 122	2	2	3	4
123 - 135	3	3	3	4
≥ 136	4	4	4	4

Child Blood Pressure Values
Boys - Age 11

Percentile of height = Less than 10%

Systolic(mm Hg)	Diastolic (mm Hg)			
	<74	74 - 77	78 - 91	≥ 92
< 113	1	2	3	4
113 - 116	2	2	3	4
117 - 129	3	3	3	4
≥ 130	4	4	4	4

Percentile of height = 10 - 24%

Systolic(mm Hg)	Diastolic (mm Hg)			
	<74	74 - 77	78 - 91	≥ 92
< 114	1	2	3	4
114 - 117	2	2	3	4
118 - 130	3	3	3	4
≥ 131	4	4	4	4

Percentile of height = 25 - 49%

Systolic(mm Hg)	Diastolic (mm Hg)			
	<75	75 - 78	79 - 92	≥ 93
< 115	1	2	3	4
115 - 118	2	2	3	4
119 - 132	3	3	3	4
≥ 133	4	4	4	4

Percentile of height = 50 - 74%

Systolic(mm Hg)	Diastolic (mm Hg)			
	<76	76 - 79	80 - 93	≥ 94
< 117	1	2	3	4
117 - 120	2	2	3	4
121 - 134	3	3	3	4
≥ 135	4	4	4	4

Percentile of height = 75 - 89%

Systolic(mm Hg)	Diastolic (mm Hg)			
	<77	77 - 80	81 - 94	≥ 95
< 119	1	2	3	4
119 - 122	2	2	3	4
123 - 135	3	3	3	4
≥ 136	4	4	4	4

Percentile of height = 90 - 94%

Systolic(mm Hg)	Diastolic (mm Hg)			
	<78	78 - 81	82 - 95	≥ 96
< 120	1	2	3	4
120 - 123	2	2	3	4
124 - 137	3	3	3	4
≥ 138	4	4	4	4

Percentile of height = 95% and higher

Systolic(mm Hg)	Diastolic (mm Hg)			
	<78	78 - 81	82 - 95	≥ 96
< 120	1	2	3	4
120 - 124	2	2	3	4
125 - 137	3	3	3	4
≥ 138	4	4	4	4

Child Blood Pressure Values
Boys - Age 12

Percentile of height = Less than 10%

Systolic(mm Hg)	Diastolic (mm Hg)			
	<74	74 - 77	78 - 91	≥ 92
< 115	1	2	3	4
115 - 118	2	2	3	4
119 - 131	3	3	3	4
≥ 132	4	4	4	4

Percentile of height = 10 - 24%

Systolic(mm Hg)	Diastolic (mm Hg)			
	<75	75 - 78	79 - 92	≥ 93
< 116	1	2	3	4
116 - 119	2	2	3	4
120 - 132	3	3	3	4
≥ 133	4	4	4	4

Percentile of height = 25 - 49%

Systolic(mm Hg)	Diastolic (mm Hg)			
	<75	75 - 79	80 - 93	≥ 94
< 118	1	2	3	4
117 - 121	2	2	3	4
122 - 134	3	3	3	4
≥ 135	4	4	4	4

Percentile of height = 50 - 74%

Systolic(mm Hg)	Diastolic (mm Hg)			
	<76	76 - 80	81 - 94	≥ 95
< 119	1	2	3	4
119 - 122	2	2	3	4
123 - 136	3	3	3	4
≥ 137	4	4	4	4

Child Blood Pressure Values
Boys - Age 12 (continued)

Percentile of height = 75 - 89%

Systolic(mm Hg)	Diastolic (mm Hg)			
	<77	77 - 81	82 - 95	≥ 96
< 120	1	2	3	4
120 - 124	2	2	3	4
125 - 138	3	3	3	4
≥ 139	4	4	4	4

Percentile of height = 90 - 94%

Systolic(mm Hg)	Diastolic (mm Hg)			
	<78	78 - 81	82 - 95	≥ 96
< 120	1	2	3	4
120 - 126	2	2	3	4
127 - 139	3	3	3	4
≥ 140	4	4	4	4

Percentile of height = 95% and higher

Systolic(mm Hg)	Diastolic (mm Hg)			
	<79	79 - 82	83 - 96	≥ 97
< 120	1	2	3	4
120 - 126	2	2	3	4
127 - 140	3	3	3	4
≥ 141	4	4	4	4

Child Blood Pressure Values
Boys - Age 13

Percentile of height = Less than 10%

Systolic(mm Hg)	Diastolic (mm Hg)			
	<75	75 - 78	79 - 92	≥ 93
< 117	1	2	3	4
117 - 120	2	2	3	4
121 - 133	3	3	3	4
≥ 134	4	4	4	4

Percentile of height = 10 - 24%

Systolic(mm Hg)	Diastolic (mm Hg)			
	<75	75 - 78	79 - 92	≥ 93
< 118	1	2	3	4
118 - 121	2	2	3	4
122 - 135	3	3	3	4
≥ 136	4	4	4	4

Percentile of height = 25 - 49%

Systolic(mm Hg)	Diastolic (mm Hg)			
	<76	76 - 79	80 - 93	≥ 94
< 120	1	2	3	4
120 - 123	2	2	3	4
124 - 136	3	3	3	4
≥ 137	4	4	4	4

Percentile of height = 50 - 74%

Systolic(mm Hg)	Diastolic (mm Hg)			
	<77	77 - 80	81 - 94	≥ 95
< 120	1	2	3	4
120 - 125	2	2	3	4
126 - 138	3	3	3	4
≥ 139	4	4	4	4

Percentile of height = 75 - 89%

Systolic(mm Hg)	Diastolic (mm Hg)			
	<78	78 - 81	82 - 95	≥ 96
< 120	1	2	3	4
120 - 127	2	2	3	4
128 - 140	3	3	3	4
≥ 141	4	4	4	4

Percentile of height = 90 - 94%

Systolic(mm Hg)	Diastolic (mm Hg)			
	<79	79 - 82	83 - 96	≥ 97
< 120	1	2	3	4
120 - 128	2	2	3	4
129 - 141	3	3	3	4
≥ 142	4	4	4	4

Percentile of height = 95% and higher

Systolic(mm Hg)	Diastolic (mm Hg)			
	<79	79 - 82	83 - 96	≥ 97
< 120	1	2	3	4
120 - 129	2	2	3	4
130 - 142	3	3	3	4
≥ 143	4	4	4	4

Child Blood Pressure Values
Boys - Age 14

Percentile of height = Less than 10%

Systolic(mm Hg)	Diastolic (mm Hg)			
	<75	75 - 79	80 - 92	≥ 93
< 120	1	2	3	4
120 - 123	2	2	3	4
124 - 136	3	3	3	4
≥ 137	4	4	4	4

Percentile of height = 10 - 24%

Systolic(mm Hg)	Diastolic (mm Hg)			
	<76	76 - 79	80 - 93	≥ 94
< 120	1	2	3	4
120 - 124	2	2	3	4
125 - 137	3	3	3	4
≥ 138	4	4	4	4

Percentile of height = 25 - 49%

Systolic(mm Hg)	Diastolic (mm Hg)			
	<77	77 - 80	81 - 94	≥ 95
< 120	1	2	3	4
120 - 126	2	2	3	4
127 - 139	3	3	3	4
≥ 140	4	4	4	4

Percentile of height = 50 - 74%

Systolic(mm Hg)	Diastolic (mm Hg)			
	<78	78 - 81	82 - 95	≥ 96
< 120	1	2	3	4
120 - 127	2	2	3	4
128 - 141	3	3	3	4
≥ 142	4	4	4	4

Child Blood Pressure Values
Boys - Age 14 (continued)

Percentile of height = 75 - 89%

Systolic(mm Hg)	Diastolic (mm Hg)			
	<79	79 - 82	83 - 96	≥ 97
< 120	1	2	3	4
120 - 129	2	2	3	4
130 - 143	3	3	3	4
≥ 144	4	4	4	4

Percentile of height = 90 - 94%

Systolic(mm Hg)	Diastolic (mm Hg)			
	<79	79 - 83	84 - 97	≥ 98
< 120	1	2	3	4
120 - 131	2	2	3	4
132 - 144	3	3	3	4
≥ 145	4	4	4	4

Percentile of height = 95% and higher

Systolic(mm Hg)	Diastolic (mm Hg)			
	<80	80 - 83	84 - 97	≥ 98
< 120	1	2	3	4
120 - 131	2	2	3	4
132 - 145	3	3	3	4
≥ 146	4	4	4	4

Child Blood Pressure Values
Boys - Age 15

Percentile of height = Less than 10%

Systolic(mm Hg)	Diastolic (mm Hg)			
	<76	76 - 80	81 - 93	≥ 94
< 120	1	2	3	4
120 - 125	2	2	3	4
126 - 139	3	3	3	4
≥ 140	4	4	4	4

Percentile of height = 10 - 24%

Systolic(mm Hg)	Diastolic (mm Hg)			
	<77	77 - 80	81 - 94	≥ 95
< 120	1	2	3	4
120 - 126	2	2	3	4
127 - 140	3	3	3	4
≥ 141	4	4	4	4

Percentile of height = 25 - 49%

Systolic(mm Hg)	Diastolic (mm Hg)			
	<78	78 - 82	83 - 95	≥ 96
< 120	1	2	3	4
120 - 128	2	2	3	4
129 - 141	3	3	3	4
≥ 142	4	4	4	4

Percentile of height = 50 - 74%

Systolic(mm Hg)	Diastolic (mm Hg)			
	<79	79 - 82	83 - 96	≥ 97
< 120	1	2	3	4
120 - 130	2	2	3	4
131 - 143	3	3	3	4
≥ 144	4	4	4	4

Percentile of height = 75 - 89%

Systolic(mm Hg)	Diastolic (mm Hg)			
	<80	80 - 83	84 - 97	≥ 98
< 120	1	2	3	4
120 - 132	2	2	3	4
133 - 145	3	3	3	4
≥ 144	4	4	4	4

Percentile of height = 90 - 94%

Systolic(mm Hg)	Diastolic (mm Hg)			
	<80	80 - 84	85 - 98	≥ 99
< 120	1	2	3	4
121 - 133	2	2	3	4
134 - 147	3	3	3	4
≥ 148	4	4	4	4

Percentile of height = 95% and higher

Systolic(mm Hg)	Diastolic (mm Hg)			
	<80	80 - 84	85 - 98	≥ 99
< 120	1	2	3	4
120 - 134	2	2	3	4
135 - 147	3	3	3	4
≥ 148	4	4	4	4

Child Blood Pressure Values
Boys - Age 16

Percentile of height = Less than 10%

Systolic(mm Hg)	Diastolic (mm Hg)			
	<78	78 - 81	82 - 95	≥ 96
< 120	1	2	3	4
120 - 128	2	2	3	4
129 - 141	3	3	3	4
≥ 142	4	4	4	4

Percentile of height = 10 - 24%

Systolic(mm Hg)	Diastolic (mm Hg)			
	<78	78 - 82	83 - 95	≥ 96
< 120	1	2	3	4
120 - 129	2	2	3	4
130 - 142	3	3	3	4
≥ 143	4	4	4	4

Percentile of height = 25 - 49%

Systolic(mm Hg)	Diastolic (mm Hg)			
	<79	79 - 82	83 - 96	≥ 97
< 120	1	2	3	4
120 - 131	2	2	3	4
132 - 144	3	3	3	4
≥ 145	4	4	4	4

Percentile of height = 50 - 74%

Systolic(mm Hg)	Diastolic (mm Hg)			
	<80	80 - 83	84 - 97	≥ 98
< 120	1	2	3	4
120 - 133	2	2	3	4
134 - 146	3	3	3	4
≥ 147	4	4	4	4

Child Blood Pressure Values
Boys - Age 16 (continued)

Percentile of height = 75 - 89%

Systolic(mm Hg)	Diastolic (mm Hg)			
	<80	80 - 84	85 - 98	≥ 99
< 120	1	2	3	4
120 - 134	2	2	3	4
135 - 148	3	3	3	4
≥ 149	4	4	4	4

Percentile of height = 90 - 94%

Systolic(mm Hg)	Diastolic (mm Hg)			
	<80	80 - 85	86 - 99	≥ 100
< 120	1	2	3	4
120 - 136	2	2	3	4
137 - 150	3	3	3	4
≥ 151	4	4	4	4

Percentile of height = 95% and higher

Systolic(mm Hg)	Diastolic (mm Hg)			
	<80	80 - 86	87 - 99	≥ 100
< 120	1	2	3	4
120 - 136	2	2	3	4
137 - 150	3	3	3	4
≥ 151	4	4	4	4

Child Blood Pressure Values
Boys - Age 17

Percentile of height = Less than 10%

Systolic(mm Hg)	Diastolic (mm Hg)			
	<80	80 - 83	84 - 97	≥ 98
< 120	1	2	3	4
120 - 130	2	2	3	4
131 - 144	3	3	3	4
≥ 145	4	4	4	4

Percentile of height = 10 - 24%

Systolic(mm Hg)	Diastolic (mm Hg)			
	<80	80 - 84	85 - 98	≥ 99
< 120	1	2	3	4
120 - 131	2	2	3	4
132 - 145	3	3	3	4
≥ 146	4	4	4	4

Percentile of height = 25 - 49%

Systolic(mm Hg)	Diastolic (mm Hg)			
	<80	80 - 85	86 - 98	≥ 99
< 120	1	2	3	4
120 - 133	2	2	3	4
134 - 146	3	3	3	4
≥ 147	4	4	4	4

Percentile of height = 50 - 74%

Systolic(mm Hg)	Diastolic (mm Hg)			
	<80	80 - 86	87 - 99	≥ 100
< 120	1	2	3	4
120 - 135	2	2	3	4
136 - 148	3	3	3	4
≥ 149	4	4	4	4

Child Blood Pressure Values
Boys - Age 17 (continued)

Percentile of height = 75 - 89%

Systolic(mm Hg)	Diastolic (mm Hg)			
	<80	80 - 86	87 - 100	≥ 101
< 120	1	2	3	4
120 - 137	2	2	3	4
148 - 150	3	3	3	4
≥ 151	4	4	4	4

Percentile of height = 90 - 94%

Systolic(mm Hg)	Diastolic (mm Hg)			
	<80	80 - 87	88 - 101	≥ 102
< 120	1	2	3	4
120 - 138	2	2	3	4
139 - 151	3	3	3	4
≥ 152	4	4	4	4

Percentile of height = 95% and higher

Systolic(mm Hg)	Diastolic (mm Hg)			
	<80	80 - 88	89 - 102	≥ 103
< 120	1	2	3	4
120 - 139	2	2	3	4
140 - 152	3	3	3	4
≥ 153	4	4	4	4

Appendix B
Child Blood Pressure References

APPENDIX B. CHILD BLOOD PRESSURE REFERENCES

Blood Pressure - Children

Referral Levels:

Level 1	(category 4)	Indicates major medical findings that warrant immediate attention by a health care provider.
Level 2	(category 3)	Indicates major medical findings that warrant attention by a health care provider within the next 2 weeks. These findings are expected to cause adverse effects within this time period and they have previously been undiagnosed, unattended, nonmanifested, or not communicated to the examinee by his or her personal health care provider.
Level 3	(categories 1 & 2)	Indicates no medical findings; minor medical findings that an examinee already knows about, and is under care for; or findings that do not require prompt attention by a medical provider.

Referral Comments for Blood Pressure (Children)

Referral Comments:

Statement for blood pressure in category 4	**Level 1 referral**	The participant's blood pressure is **very high** based on the 1996 update of the Task Force Report on High Blood Pressure in Children and Adolescents.*
Statement for blood pressure in category 3	**Level 2 referral**	The participant's blood pressure is **high** based on the 1996 update of the Task Force Report on High Blood Pressure in Children and Adolescents.*
Statement for blood pressure in category 2	**Level 3 no referral**	The participant's blood pressure is **normal but at the high end of normal** based on the 1996 update of the Task Force Report on High Blood Pressure in Children and Adolescents.*
Statement for blood pressure in category 1	**Level 3 no referral**	The participant's blood pressure is **normal** based on the 1996 update of the Task Force Report on High Blood Pressure in Children and Adolescents.*

Report of Findings Comments:

- Category 4   Your child's blood pressure today is **<u>very high</u>**.

- Category 3   Your child's blood pressure today is **<u>high</u>**.

- Category 2   Your child's blood pressure today is **<u>normal but at the high end of the normal range</u>**.

- Category 1   Your child's blood pressure today is **<u>normal</u>**.

* National High Blood Pressure Education Program Working Group on Hypertension Control in Children and Adolescents. Update on the 1987 Task Force Report on High Blood Pressure in Children and Adolescents: A Working Group Report from the National High Blood Pressure Education Program. *Pediatrics*. 1996;11:649-658.

Appendix C
Adult Blood Pressure Reference Tables

APPENDIX C. ADULT BLOOD PRESSURE REFERENCE TABLES

Referral levels for adult blood pressure[1]

Systolic	Diastolic				
	<80	80-89	90-99	100-119	>/=120
<120	1	2	3	4	5
120-139	2	2	3	4	5
140-159	3	3	3	4	5
160-209	4	4	4	4	5
>/= 210	5	5	5	5	5

[1] **Based on the Seventh Report of the Joint National Committee on the Prevention, Detection, Evaluation, and Treatment of High Blood Pressure. NIH Publication, 2003.**

Blood Pressure Referral Levels, Category, and Action Required

Referral Level	BP Category	Physician Guideline Referral Action
Level 1	Category 5	Indicates major medical findings that warrant immediate attention by a health care provider.
Level 2	Categories 3 & 4	Indicates major medical findings that warrant attention by a health care provider within the next 2 weeks. These findings are expected to cause adverse effects within this time period and they have previously been undiagnosed, unattended, nonmanifested, or not communicated to the examinee by his or her personal health care provider.
Level 2	Category 2	Indicates prehypertensive blood pressure, minor medical findings that an examinee already knows about and is under care for, or findings that do not require prompt attention by a medical provider within a month.
Level 3	Category 1	Indicates no abnormal medical findings.

Table of Blood Pressure Report of Findings Comments – English and Spanish

Report of Findings level	Report of Findings Message - English	Report of Findings Message - Spanish
1	Your blood pressure today is within the normal range, based on the Seventh Report of the Joint National Committee on the Prevention, Detection, Evaluation, and Treatment of High Blood Pressure. NIH Publication, 2003.	Su presión de sangre hoy está dentro del rango normal. Basado en el Séptimo Informe del Comité Conjunto Nacional de Prevención, Detección, Evaluación y Tratamiento de la Alta Presión Sanguínea. Publicación del NIH, 2003.
2	Your blood pressure today is above normal and is in the prehypertensive range, based on the Seventh Report of the Joint National Committee on the Prevention, Detection, Evaluation, and Treatment of High Blood Pressure. NIH Publication, 2003.	Su presión de sangre hoy es por encima de lo normal y está dentro del rango de prehipertensión. Basado en el Séptimo Informe del Comité Conjunto Nacional de Prevención, Detección, Evaluación y Tratamiento de la Alta Presión Sanguínea. Publicación del NIH, 2003.
3	Your blood pressure today is high, based on the Seventh Report of the Joint National Committee on the Prevention, Detection, Evaluation, and Treatment of High Blood Pressure. NIH Publication, 2003.	Su presión de sangre hoy es alta. Basado en el Séptimo Informe del Comité Conjunto Nacional de Prevención, Detección, Evaluación y Tratamiento de la Alta Presión Sanguínea. Publicación del NIH, 2003.
4	Your blood pressure today is very high, based on the Seventh Report of the Joint National Committee on the Prevention, Detection, Evaluation, and Treatment of High Blood Pressure. NIH Publication, 2003.	Su presión de sangre hoy es muy alta. Basado en el Séptimo Informe del Comité Conjunto Nacional de Prevención, Detección, Evaluación y Tratamiento de la Alta Presión Sanguínea. Publicación del NIH, 2003.
5	Your blood pressure today is severely high.	Su presión de sangre hoy es severamente alta.

(Note: ROF level number 5 should **not** have the NIH Publication referenced.

Report of Findings Comments:

- Category 5 - Your blood pressure today is **severely high**.

- Category 4 - Your blood pressure today is **very high**.

- Category 3 - Your blood pressure today is **high**.

- Category 2 - Your blood pressure today is above normal **and in the prehypertensive range.**

- Category 1 - Your blood pressure today is **within the normal range.**

Appendix D

STD Information Sheets and Role Plays

MEC INFORMATION SHEETS

INFECTIONS WITH HERPES SIMPLEX VIRUS TYPE 2

Mode of infection

- Almost always sexual

Laboratory assay used in NHANES

- Type specific immunodot assay using sera, which measures antibodies specific for HSV-2. This test result is an indicator of past infection.

Frequency

- Approximately 1 in 10 adolescents

- Increases with age among white adults to over 1 in 4 adults

- Increases with age among black adults to over 1 in 2 adults

Location of the initial infection and of symptoms

- Women

    - Skin around the vagina, urethra, and rectum

    - Skin of inner thighs and on the buttocks

    - In the vagina and on the cervix

- Men

    - Skin on and around the penis

    - Skin of inner thighs

    - Rectum and skin around the rectum and on the buttocks

Latent infection

- Most of the time, the virus remains dormant in nerve cells connected to the lower spinal cord.

- Symptoms occur when the virus begins to replicate in skin cells around the nerve endings.

Symptoms of uncomplicated infection

- Most infected individuals report no symptoms.

- Blisters that break to form multiple small tender sores that heal spontaneously within a week.

- Episodes recur with highly variable frequency, symptom-free intervals ranging from days to months.

Complications

- Occasionally, the sores are sufficiently painful to interfere with urination.

- Rarely, infection of the brain occurs.

- Rarely, babies born to infected women contract serious infections.

Diagnosis

- Blood tests to detect antibody.

  - In NHANES, a special blood test is used that is not yet available to most physicians. The blood test detects antibody and is usually correct, but no test is 100% accurate.

  - Physicians can order blood tests, but they do not reliably distinguish between the type 2 herpes simplex virus infection and type 1 infection that is the infection that most commonly causes fever blisters of the mouth and is not usually sexually transmitted.

- Cultures and other tests detect the virus in blisters and sores, except during the later stage of healing.

- Frequently, the blisters, sores, and history of recurrences are characteristic, and the physician requires no laboratory test to make the diagnosis.

NOTE: Except by using the NHANES type of blood test, the infection cannot be detected unless blisters or ulcers are present.

Treatment

- No treatment is curative.

- Antiviral drugs suppress symptoms, which usually recur after the drug is stopped.

- Treatment of each recurrence, separately, is not usually worthwhile, because healing occurs before the drug can act.

Preventing infection of others

- Transmission-related factors

  - Intimate, usually sexual, contact is required.

  - Infected individuals are most infectious when they have sores, but they most often infect others when they are asymptomatic.

  - Infected individuals, who never have symptoms, often shed herpes virus, but how many are infectious is unknown.

- Prevention measures should be taken, but they are not entirely effective.

  - Visit a physician, who can help the infected person determine when a herpes outbreak is occurring.

  - Avoid intercourse during outbreaks.

  - Use condoms.

  - Make sex partners aware of need for preventive measures and residual risks.

MEC INFORMATION SHEETS

INFECTIONS WITH HUMAN IMMUNODEFICIENCY VIRUS

Mode of infection

- Sexual transmission and percutaneous blood exposure (IV drug use, needle sticks in health care workers, etc.).

Laboratory assay used in NHANES

- Serum is screened for HIV-1 antibody using an FDA-licensed enzyme immuno assay kit. Repeatedly reactive specimens are then tested by an FDA-licensed Western blot assay.

Frequency

- Approximately 3 in 1,000 adults

- Approximately 2 in 1,000 white adults

- Approximately 11 in 1,000 black adults

- Approximately 4 in 1,000 Mexican American adults

Diagnosis

- Blood tests to detect antibody

Incubation (infection to AIDS diagnosis)

- Median 8-10 years in untreated individual, but varies by age.

- Treatment with HAART (highly active antiretroviral therapy) is altering the median incubation time.

Treatment

- HAART, if given early, can slow or stop disease progression.

- Treatment of opportunistic infections as they occur.

Preventing infection of others

- Condom use has been demonstrated to be effective against transmission.

- Only abstinence or monogamous relationship (between two HIV negative partners) is totally effective in preventing exposure.

This page is intentionally blank.

Reproductive Health/Sexually Transmitted Diseases

STD	Symptoms	Treatment	Things to Know
HIV/AIDS (virus)	None or mild flu-like symptoms early in infection. With onset of AIDS many years after infection, persistent cough, unexplained weight loss, diarrhea, fever, etc.	Treatment is available to slow or stop disease progression. Many serious AIDS-related infections can be prevented by medications.	Early treatment can delay serious complications. Treatment of pregnant HIV positive women can reduce transmission to the baby.
Gonorrhea (clap, drip, GC) (bacterium)	Most women and many men have no symptoms. **Women**: Abnormal vaginal discharge, burning on urination or lower abdominal pain. **Men**: Discharge of pus from penis; burning on urination.	Can be cured with antibiotics. Sex partners need to be treated.	If not treated, can lead to more serious problems. Gonorrhea can lead to infertility in women. A mother can pass the infection on to her baby.
Chlamydia (bacterium)	Most women and many men have no symptoms. **Women**: Mild or no symptoms; vaginal discharge; burning on urination or lower abdominal pain. **Men**: Discharge from penis; burning or pain on urination.	Can be cured with antibiotics. Sex partners need to be treated.	If not treated, Chlamydia can lead to more serious problems. Reproductive organs can be damaged (Pelvic Inflammatory Disease). A mother can pass the infection on to her baby.

Reproductive Health/Sexually Transmitted Diseases (continued)

STD	Symptoms	Treatment	Things to Know
Genital Herpes (virus)	Most women and many men have no symptoms. Painful blisters. Painful urination. Swollen glands in groin area and fever.	Herpes cannot be cured but medication can reduce symptoms.	Symptoms disappear and may recur at any time. Infected persons are most likely to transmit the infection when they have symptoms, but they can also transmit when they don't have symptoms. In rare instances a mother can give herpes to her infant during childbirth.
Bacterial Vaginosis (BV) (bacterial growth)	**Women:** Most women have no symptoms. Others have a gray, thin vaginal discharge with an odor.	Can be cured with antibiotics. May recur and require repeat or long-term treatment.	If not treated, can lead to more serious problems. It is very important for pregnant women to get treated. Women who have never had sexual intercourse can get BV.
Trichomonas (protozoan)	Many women have no symptoms. Some women have a yellow gray or green vaginal discharge with an odor. Burning, irritation of the vaginal area.	Can be cured with antibiotics. Sex partners need to be treated.	It is very important for pregnant women to get treated.
Syphilis (bacterium)	Many women and men have no symptoms. Painless ulcers in the genital area. New infection may produce sore genitals, an unusual rash, fever, or swollen lymph nodes.	Can be cured with antibiotics.	If not treated, syphilis can lead to long-term health problems including heart disease and nerve problems. It is very important for pregnant women to get treated.

Reproductive Health/Sexually Transmitted Diseases (continued)

STD	Symptoms	Treatment	Things to Know
Human Papillomavirus (virus)	Many people have no symptoms. Symptoms and signs of infection are genital warts, abnormal Pap smear, cervical lesions, and cervical cancer.	HPV is not cured with medicine, but symptoms can be treated.	Some types of HPV are linked to cervical cancer, others to genital warts. HPV infection can resolve on its own.

For information and/or test results, call the NHANES Health Educator: 1-888-301-2360, Monday – Friday 9 AM to 6 PM Eastern Standard Time.

Your participation is giving researchers valuable information about the number of people in this country who are infected with sexually transmitted diseases (STDs). In order to get accurate numbers, we test all survey participants in your age group, even if you are not at risk for getting these diseases.

Your test results are completely confidential and will not be reported to your family, employers, insurers, or intimate contacts. Your doctor can receive results only with your permission. Test results are given only to you. Four weeks after the exam, you may call our health educator toll free at 1-888-301-2360 for your STD results (including HIV testing for those aged 18-49 years). You must provide your password before any results are given out. Please make sure you remember this password when you call. If a health problem is identified, you will be told how to get evaluated and treated.

Other phone numbers you can call:
National STD Hotline
1-800-227-8922

and the AIDS Hotline
1-800-342-AIDS

This page is intentionally blank.

ROLE PLAY—SCENARIO 1:

Client

Sam is a 45-year-old divorcé who left his former wife about a year ago. He was married for 20 years and has two children. He has never had an STD, just a urinary tract infection once. He has heard much about HIV/AIDS and is worried how to date safely in the '90s. He is a sample person for the NHANES survey and is willing to be tested for STDs. He is in general good health and looks forward to developing a new romantic relationship.

Counselor

You will be counseling Sam a 45-year-old divorcé who has recently rejoined the dating scene. He is worried about HIV/AIDS and wants to become romantically involved again but safely. He is not very aware of the various types of STDs and the associated symptoms.

You will need to provide a smooth segue into this part of the physician's exam. Discuss the purpose of testing for STD/HIV and why these special tests have a different mechanism for reporting. Assure confidentiality of the survey and test results. If asked, explain and educate Sam on the various STDs, risk behaviors associated with transmission, complications, testing methods, and possible treatments available if found to be infected. In closing, you will arrange for Sam to call to obtain his results if he wishes, in a confidential manner.

Observer

As the observer, you are not to interrupt or engage in the counseling session. Take side notes of the counselor's ability to cover the major points listed:

- Smooth segue into STD/HIV component of physician's exam;
- Assure confidential manner of testing and obtaining results;

- When asked, explain the various types of STDs, risk behaviors, testing methods, associated symptoms, and treatments available if found to be infected; and

- Mechanisms for client to obtain results.

Did the counselor listen to the client to assess risk and knowledge level of the client about STDs?

Did the counselor use open-ended questions to better assess the client's level of understanding?

Did the client appear to understand the level of communication that the counselor was speaking from?

Did the counselor adequately cover the bullets highlighted above?

ROLE PLAY—SCENARIO 2:

Client

Julie is a 19-year-old college student. She has never had an STD and has recently becme sexually involved with her boyfriend, Bob, whom she has been dating for 1 year. She has heard about STDs but is not very familiar with symptoms or ways to be tested for them. She is in general good health and looks forward to a happy and healthy future with Bob when she finishes college.

Counselor

You will be counseling Julie, a 19-year-old college student, who has recently become sexually active with her boyfriend Bob. She is not very aware of the various types of STDs and the associated symptoms.

You will need to provide a smooth segue into this part of the physician's exam. Discuss the purpose of testing for STD/HIV and why these special tests have a different mechanism for reporting. Assure confidentiality of the survey and tests methods involved. If asked, explain and educate Julie on the various STDs, risk behaviors associated with transmission, sequelae, testing methods, and possible treatments available if found to be infected. In closing, you will arrange for Julie to call to obtain her results if she wishes, in a confidential manner.

Observer

As the observer you are not to interrupt or engage in the counseling session. Take side notes of the counselor's ability to cover the major points listed:

- Smooth segue into STD/HIV component of physician's exam;

- Assure confidential manner of testing and obtaining results;

- When asked, explain the various types of STDs, risk behaviors, testing methods, associated symptoms, and treatments available if found to be infected; and

- Mechanisms for client to obtain results.

Did the counselor listen to the client and address specific questions about STDs?

Did the counselor use open-ended questions to better assess the client's level of understanding?

Did the client appear to understand the level of communication that the counselor was speaking from?

Did the counselor adequately cover the bullets highlighted above?

ROLE PLAY—SCENARIO 3:

Client

Jack Williams is 42-years-old and married with two children. He has been married for 12 years and works for a new car dealer. He spent 4 years in the Navy and was once infected with gonorrhea while on leave in Japan. While in the Navy he had to attend presentations about STD/HIV and is familiar with their symptoms and treatment.

Counselor

You will be talking to Jack about the NHANES project and seeking his permission to test him for STDs and HIV.

You will provide a smooth segue into this part of the examination, assure him that everything is confidential, and explain the test procedures. Explain why he is being tested, the purpose of the project, and what your role is with the project. If Jack agrees to be tested, make arrangements for him to call back for his test results.

Observer

Do not interrupt the session. Take notes of the following:

- Smooth segue into STD/HIV component of physician's exam;

- Assure confidential manner of testing and obtaining results;

- When asked, explain the various types of STDs, risk behaviors, testing methods, associated symptoms, and treatments available if found to be infected; and

- Mechanisms for client to obtain results.

Did the counselor address the above checklist?

Did the counselor address questions the client may have asked?

Appendix E

Procedures for Handling Mercury Manometers

APPENDIX E

PROCEDURES FOR HANDLING MERCURY MANOMETERS

E.1   Background

The elemental mercury in the Baum mercury manometer is encased in a closed system composed of a glass tube and reservoir, and unless exposed to the atmosphere, is harmless. Elemental mercury is a shiny, silver-gray metal that is a liquid at room temperature and which gives off a toxic vapor when exposed to the atmosphere. Although it is less toxic than the organic compound of methylmercury, elemental mercury, $Hg(0)$, can cause tremors, gingivitis, and excitability when vapors are directly inhaled over a long period of time. Temperature, ventilation, and sunlight affect the level of the vapor's concentration, and the vapors can permeate the skin surface and are easily inhaled. If elemental mercury is ingested, it is absorbed relatively slowly and may pass through the digestive system without causing damage

According to the manufacturer, the elemental mercury used in Baum manometers is safely contained in the reservoir and Mylar® Clad Calibrated Cartridge glass tube. Since February of 1995, Baum has applied several layers of very strong and crystal clear Mylar® film to the glass tubes, which strengthen the tube and maintain its structural integrity even if the inner glass is broken. The Mylar® sheath ends close to the tube's top end, and a fingernail can detect the change in the tube's outer diameter, which indicates that this tube has the Mylar film.

A mercury sphygmomanometer should be handled with extreme care. The instrument should not be dropped or treated in any way that could result in damage to the manometer. Regular quality control checks are conducted to ensure that there are no leaks from the inflation system and that the manometer has not been damaged so as to cause a loss of mercury. The Baum mercury manometers are designed to minimize mercury releases from its closed system; however, there are two ways in which mercury can be released from the manometers.

The glass tube release lever at the top of the wall mounted manometers is one potential source of mercury spillage. If this lever is inadvertently flipped back while the instrument is upright on the wall, the glass tube is released and the mercury spills out of the bottom of the tube. The lever should only be moved by a service technician when the sphygmomanometer is removed from the wall and lying on its right side. Baum has added a safety feature to this release lever, with the addition of a "set screw" that prevents an accidental movement of the lever without a tool. If the unit has not been retrofitted with the "set screw" during routine maintenance, a safety modification, a "lever lock" is available free of charge from Baum. The "lever lock" is simply a small piece of metal bent at a 90 degree angle, which is easily slipped behind the lever to immobilize it. Once installed, the lever lock can be removed with a screwdriver. Spills are prevented because users cannot remove the lever lock without some effort; the lock simply eliminates the potential for anyone to idly flip the release lever.

The second manner in which mercury could be released is if the glass tube is damaged in some way. With the application of Mylar® to the glass tube, the incidence of glass tube damage has been drastically reduced. According to Baum, the mercury within the tube is contained within the Mylar coating.

E.2 Mercury Sphygmomanometer Procedures

The mercury devices maintained in the physician component are:

- One (1) wall-mounted unit model 33 Baum manometer;

- One (1) backup wall-mounted unit; and

- One (1) backup desktop unit.

At this time, physicians alone have the responsibility for installing the wall-mounted manometers, and this includes the blood pressure methodology study room.

The backup units should be kept in boxes in sealed plastic double bags in their own dedicated plastic bins.

All mercury manometers are periodically sent for cleaning and maintenance to Baum. The wall manometers in use should be taken down and sent back to the warehouse twice per year for servicing following the last day of exams prior to the summer and winter holiday vacations. Install the backup manometer, and send an inventory UFO that alerts the warehouse manager to send a replacement wall-mounted manometer to the field.

If a defect or irregularity is observed during a routine QC check, never attempt to repair the equipment yourself. Notify the MEC manager and package the manometer in preparation for shipping to the NHANES warehouse. The MEC manager will inform the warehouse manager that a replacement backup manometer is required. Packing, shipping, and installing these manometers require specific procedures to be followed.

E.2.1   Wall-Mounted Unit Model 33

Unpacking and mounting the unit

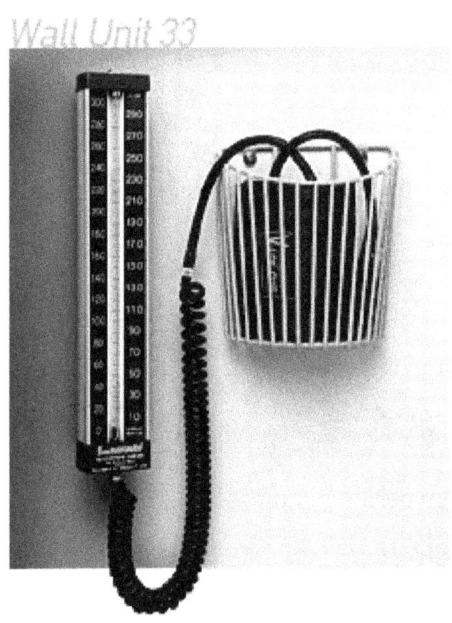

The manometers are sent to the MEC in a sealed box, and are stored on the MEC in dedicated plastic bins. The wall mount bracket is in place on the wall in the physician component room, as well as the blood pressure methodology room.

1.   Remove the manometer from the box. ****IMPORTANT: Save the box—do not discard****; the box is required for safely storing and shipping the manometer back to the warehouse.

2.   Carefully inspect the outer bag for mercury droplets. If no mercury is seen, remove contents from the outer bag.

3. Inspect inner bag for mercury droplets. If no mercury is seen, open bag and remove manometer.

4. To remove the blue shipping seal, place the instrument on its side and hold it securely. Grasp the blue shipping seal and pull it out. Important: you must remove the blue shipping seal before the instrument is mounted on the wall or pressurized.

5. Inspect the cartridge tube release lever located at the top of the manometer casing in front of the swivel screw. This lever releases the glass tube cartridge, *which should never be released under any circumstances on the MEC*. If the lever is not secured with a factory installed "set screw," Baum has supplied us with L-shaped lever lock inserts designed to prevent tampering with the cartridge tube release lever and accidental release of mercury. See the following section for Lever Lock insertion instructions.

6. Remove the red cap from the metal connector at the bottom of the instrument. *******IMPORTANT: Save the red cap—do not discard******; the red cap is required for storing and shipping the manometer. Tape the red cap to the box, and place the box inside the plastic bags.

7. Attach the instrument onto the mounting bracket attached to the wall. Tighten the chrome plated swivel screw at the top of the bracket, securing the manometer to the bracket with a flat head screw driver.

8. Attach the coiled Extendex® tubing to the metal connector at the bottom of the instrument.

9. Note the serial number located at the top right face of the manometer, just above the number 290, and give this to the MEC manager to be entered into the equipment tracking system.

10. Continue with equipment QC procedures.

Lever Lock Insertion Instructions:

Although Baumanometer wall units sold in the last few years come equipped with a glass tube release lever secured with a "set screw" that keeps the lever in place, older models without these set screws are still common. While the manometers that are being sent to Baum for servicing return with the set screws, the survey does have the older models that do not have this safety feature. See the following instructions for inserting the lever locks provided by Baum.

Purpose

To prevent tampering with the cartridge tube release lever and accidental release of mercury.

Lever Lock Insertion Instructions (after-factory safety enhancement)

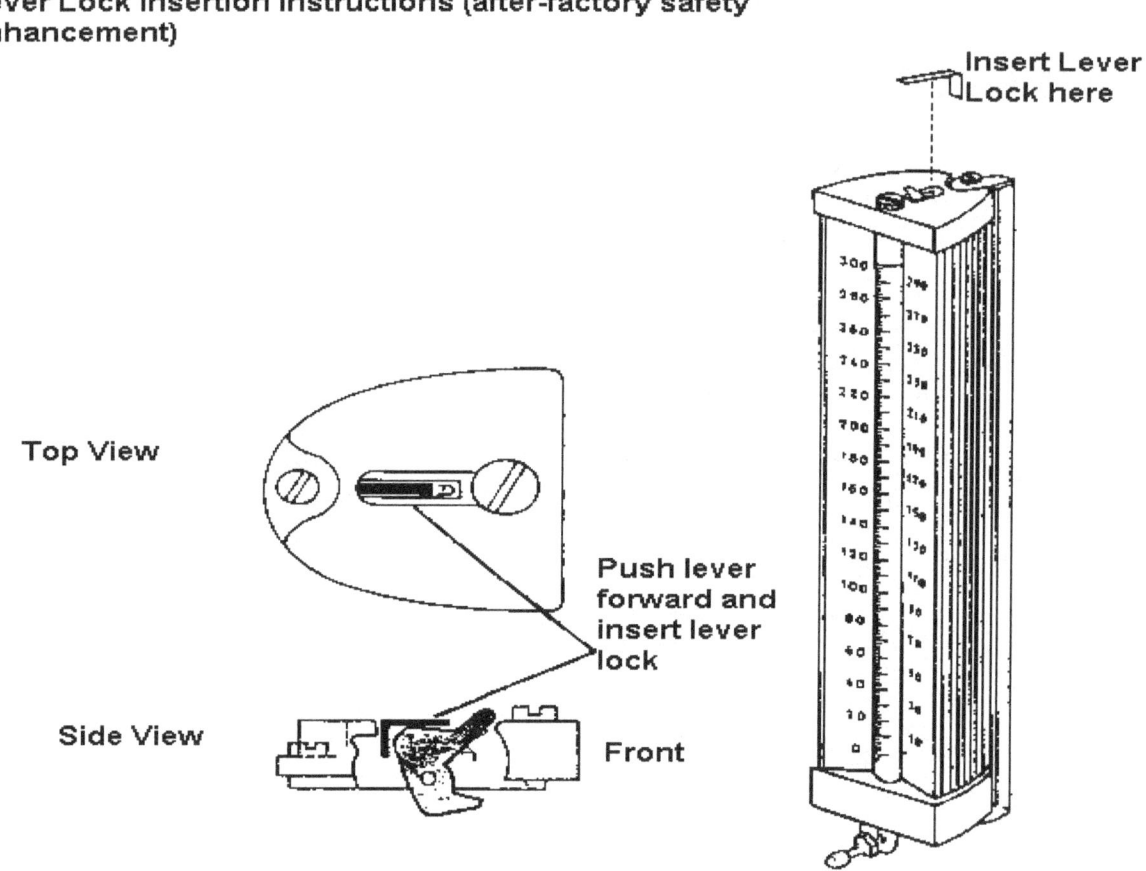

Teardown Procedures for Wall-Mounted Manometers

Installed wall-mounted manometers:

The installed wall-mounted manometers are left in place during MEC transport.

1.   Complete the end-of-stand QC procedures for the manometer.

2.   Observe that the swivel screw at the top of the manometer that secures the manometer to the wall bracket is sufficiently tight.

3.   Place the cushions provided securely around the manometer.

Backup wall-mounted manometers:

1.   Keep the manometer in the packing--double plastic bags and box.

2.   Store in the bin used for the manometers and pack in the black storage box.

3.   Place in storage container in physician's room for transport to next stand.

*****Important: Do not store the mercury-containing manometers in the belly compartment during transport.*****

Packing Wall-Mounted Manometers for Shipping

1.   Remove the coiled Extendex ® tubing from the instrument.

2.   Attach the red cap firmly to the tubing connector on the instrument to seal.

3.   Check that the lever lock, if needed, is in place on top of the instrument. If not, see attached instructions for inserting a lever lock.

4.   Remove the instrument from the wall unit.

5.   Place instrument in a plastic bag and seal closed with adhesive tape. Repeat this process with another plastic bag so that the unit is double bagged.

6.   Wrap manometer box with bubble wrap.

7.   Place the wrapped manometer into a box for shipping.

8.   Give the boxed manometer to the MEC manager.

9.   The MEC manager will enter the transfer of the equipment from the MEC to the warehouse in the equipment tracking system, and send the unit to the warehouse.

E.2.2   Desk-top Mercury Manometer

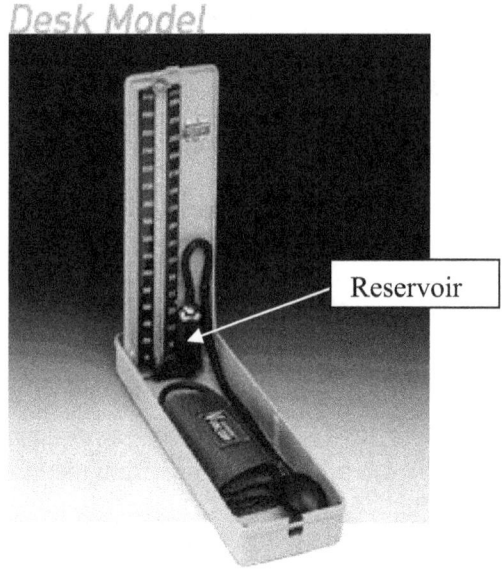

One Baum Desk Model mercury manometer is maintained as a backup manometer in the physician component. It is intended for use as a backup instrument for both the physician component as well as the blood pressure methodology study. The desk model weighs 2.7 pounds. Unlike the wall-mounted Baum manometer, the desk model does not require a safety enhancement like the lever lock.

Unpacking Desk Model Manometers:

1.   Open box and remove manometer.

2.   Carefully inspect outer bag for mercury droplets. If no mercury is seen, open bag and remove contents.

3.   Carefully inspect the inner bag for mercury droplets. If no mercury is seen, open bag and remove the manometer box.

4.   Open manometer and place upright on table.

5.   Remove red cap from reservoir and reconnect tubing.

Packing Desk Model Manometer:

1. Tilt manometer onto reservoir-side. Mercury should be contained in reservoir.

2. Remove tubing from top of mercury reservoir.

3. Place red cap firmly on reservoir opening while manometer is on its side.

4. Stand manometer up, and close the unit.

5. Place instrument in a plastic bag and seal closed, then fold the end of the bag over and seal it with adhesive tape. Repeat this process with another plastic bag so that the unit is double bagged.

6. Wrap manometer box with bubble wrap.

7. Place the wrapped manometer into a box for shipping.

8. Place in storage container in physician's room for transport to next stand.